A *Holistt*
Preventi
and Creating a Healthier,
More Vibrant Future

Don't Let the Memories Fade

Based on the *Eight Weeks to a Better Brain* Program

Kate Kunkel

This book is dedicated to my mom
and to my grandmothers -
three amazing women who taught me
the meaning of strength.

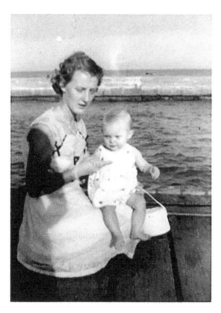

Inez and Kate 1958

Table of Contents

Introduction

Ten years ago, when my mom was starting to show signs of Alzheimer's, I knew nothing about this affliction. I had no idea that her personality changes were the beginning of a terrible journey upon which she was about to embark. I never imagined that the force of nature that was my mother could ever succumb to such devastation.

It was insidious. First it was occasional loss of words and garbled sentences. Then she became withdrawn and even lost interest in the dolls that had been her life. She eventually became combative and could not sleep, pacing the floor, looking for things she could not find.

Doctors were no help, saying it was inevitable that she would steadily decline. They said there was nothing we could do.

As I look back on it, I realize that even if I had known then what I know now, I might not have been able to help Mom because by the time we realized what was happening, her Alzheimer's was too far advanced. But I often wonder, if I had known the warning signs, could we have delayed her decline? Maybe those last years could have at least been more pleasant for her. And maybe we would have been able to say goodbye.

Mom passed away in December of 2019. The last months of her life were terrible. In the throes of her dementia, Mom developed cancer again, and there was no possibility of treatment because she was unable to comprehend what that meant. She was so agitated that her doctors couldn't even examine her properly.

Mom did not die peacefully. She was afraid and she was in pain. And she couldn't even express her pain or fear because she no longer had the words. It is a terrible way to die.

But she is only one of millions who suffer and die with this disease every moment. One in three seniors in North America dies with Alzheimer's or some other form of dementia, and this beast kills more people than breast cancer and prostate cancer combined.

We've been told that so many people are succumbing because the population is aging. But that just does not account for the increase in numbers, and it's not the luck of the genetic draw.

After my mom received her diagnosis, I began digging and found out that our environment, our lifestyles, the food we eat, and the water we drink are all contributing to this epidemic. When I learned this I started getting angry.

Why wasn't this information out there in the mainstream? Why didn't the doctors who were treating my mom know this, and why didn't they recommend ways we could get a handle on it before her disease became too advanced? Why didn't these professionals, who work with dementia patients every day, know what I was learning? How could they miss the hundreds – no, thousands – of published research papers available around the globe?

Because they aren't trained to look beyond the pharmaceutical solution for anything, especially Alzheimer's and other dementias. They are told, and believe, that dementia cannot be prevented or reversed.

But that is simply not true.

Dementia can be prevented, and in many cases,
if you catch it early enough, it can also be reversed!

By the time Mom was losing her ability to communicate, I was also starting to have memory issues. Everybody said it was just stress, but I was terrified. I was desperate to avoid the path my mother was traveling, so I made it my business to learn everything I could about dementia.

I learned about inflammation and insulin resistance and stress and how sleep deprivation and toxic cleaning products can wreak havoc on your brain. I also learned that mindfully listening to music and engaging in a meditation practice can save your brain. I got to work figuring out what steps I needed to take to save my own brain and become healthier. These lifestyle changes have been life-changers.

I don't forget why I walked into the room now, and I don't lose my keys. I've lost 40 pounds and feel stronger and have more energy than I did when I was in my 30s. I remember appointments and don't struggle for words.

So now I'm on a mission. I'm committed to spreading the word that nobody else ever has to suffer like Mom did. In workshops and programs and now in this book, I'm sharing the exact things I did, and that you can do, to not only protect your memories and your brain but also boost your energy level and improve your overall health.

My fervent wish is that everyone understands this one thing: It is never too early to look after your brain, but it can get too late. We should all assume that we are at risk and do everything we can as soon as we can to protect our memories and our future.

How to Use This Book

In the first half of this book you'll learn the risk factors and the warning signs. You'll learn where you might be vulnerable and where and why you should be focusing your efforts. At the end of the book are footnotes with links to papers and articles that support the information. If you like to geek out on research, this is your space!

Beginning in chapter 11, I describe the *Eight Weeks to a Better Brain* program along with the supporting information that will help you integrate the three pillars of health – body, mind, and spirit – to make these amazing improvements.

Finally, to make things as easy as possible, in the appendix I include recipes, sample meal plans, meditations, and references to resources that will help you get started right away.

You can hop to chapter 11 any time to get started, but please be sure to read the first 10 chapters at some point to understand why you're doing everything you do. That will help you maintain your resolve to fully embrace this wonderful lifestyle.

Let's get started!

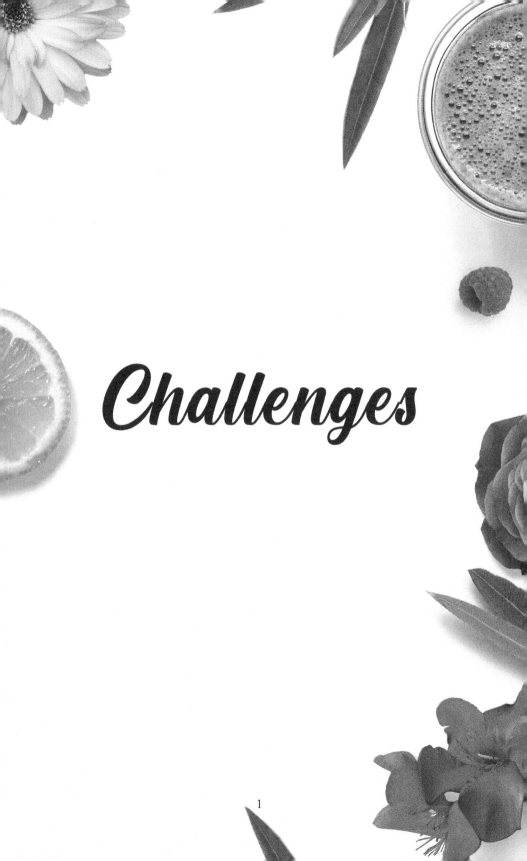

Challenges

Chapter 1

What Is This Thing Called Dementia?

Do not believe it when someone tells you,
"It can't be helped."
I'm here to tell you it can.
But you have to work at it. Just like anything else worth fighting for.

Alzheimer's Disease or Dementia?

You've probably heard *Alzheimer's disease (Alzheimer's, or AD)* and *dementia* used interchangeably. But they are not the same.

Dementia is an umbrella term for syndromes that have many different symptoms, including forgetfulness, difficulty with complex tasks, confusion about time and space, and much more.

Alzheimer's disease is the most well-known and common form of dementia. Everyone with Alzheimer's has dementia, but not everyone with dementia has Alzheimer's disease.

Alzheimer's disease exists when one protein in the brain, beta-amyloid, (often just called amyloid), reaches an abnormal level. It forms plaques that collect between neurons and disrupts the function of cells in the brain. Another protein that's involved is called tau. When it reaches an abnormal level, it forms neurofibrillary tangles inside the neurons. Eventually these tangles block the neurons' transport system so they cannot communicate. The presence of these tangles and plaques is what defines Alzheimer's. However, some people have a brain full of tangles and have no cognitive problems, while others with none have full-blown dementia.

I discuss later in the book why and how these proteins develop (hint: lifestyle choices), but it's important to understand that while they can wreak havoc on memory and brain function, they are not the evil invaders that the pharmaceutical industry has demonized. According to several researchers, including Dr. Dale Bredesen,[1] one of the preeminent dementia researchers, these proteins are normal protective responses to inflammation, exposure to toxins or unfriendly bacteria, and/or a lack of important nutrients. Their presence means your defense mechanism has run amok.

For some people, an overcharged immune system leads to a disease like multiple sclerosis or rheumatoid arthritis. For others it leads to Alzheimer's. But the immune system is mostly just doing its job. It is responding to inflammation, infection, stress, or toxicity that threatens the health of the brain.

You've also probably heard that if you have a genetic predisposition to Alzheimer's, you're doomed. That is simply not true. In fact, many people who carry the gene (APOE4) do not develop Alzheimer's, and many who do not have the gene do develop the disease.[2]

Another form of dementia, frontotemporal, also has a genetic component, but recent research shows that it, too, can be thwarted by adopting lifestyle changes[3] including good nutrition, exercise, and stress-management techniques.

Stats and Facts

As of 2018, Alzheimer's disease officially ranked as the sixth leading cause of death in the United States. But recent estimates are placing it in third place, just behind cancer and heart disease, as a cause of death for older people.

Dementia in all its forms already plagues more than 5.8 million Americans and over half a million Canadians. About 50 million people worldwide are suffering from dementia now, and the total number is projected to reach 82 million in 2030 and 152 million in 2050.

It's interesting that India, which has a population of 1.4 billion, has only four million people affected by this devastating disease. Compare this to the U.S., which has a population of just 327.2 million. Even accounting for lower life expectancy, Indians are less than one-third as likely to die with dementia.

Here are some other interesting statistics: According to the latest World Health Organization (WHO) data published in 2017, the death rate for dementia in the U.S. is 44.41 per 100,000 people. Compare this to my adopted country, Ecuador, where only 4.47 people in 100,000 died from dementia in 2017. There are many theories about why the rate in Ecuador is so much lower, but these differences in death rates indicate to me that something about lifestyle differences between cultures must be the factor.

So what's the difference between the U.S. and India? The lowest rates of Alzheimer's are in areas of India that are predominantly vegetarian.

In most areas of Ecuador, where I live, fruits and vegetables are cheap and plentiful. Sure, there is some encroachment of sugary sodas and fast food chains, but most food is local and fresh. I literally cannot remember the last time I ate a packaged item here.

That tells us that, contrary to "official" sources that assert that dementia is the only disease of the 10 leading causes of deaths in Europe and North America that cannot be cured, prevented, or slowed, there are ways to prevent it. Not only are there ways to prevent it, there are also treatments that have been successful in reversing the symptoms.

The Many Faces of Dementia

Dementia is not a specific disease. It's a syndrome with a wide range of symptoms that impact a person's ability to independently perform everyday activities. There are many different types and causes of dementia, including:

Alzheimer's disease. There are three main stages of the disease, each with its own symptoms. Symptoms generally begin with having less interest in work and social activities, less energy and drive to do things, forgetting recent conversations, and having trouble putting thoughts into words. As the disease progresses, patients have trouble sleeping, they often wander, their speech might ramble, and they can get lost in familiar places. They also get angry or upset easily, sometimes lashing out at family members or caregivers, accusing them of stealing or trying to hurt them. In later stages they are usually incontinent and can even forget how to eat on their own.

Vascular dementia.[4] This is a common post-stroke problem and the second most common form of dementia. While the risk of developing it depends on the location and severity of the stroke, age, sex, and family history are also factors.

The same factors that contribute to strokes also contribute to Alzheimer's and other dementias. According to a 2012 study, for adults over 65, stroke is a risk factor for dementia and dementia is a risk factor for stroke.

Symptoms of vascular dementia include difficulty with focus, organization, and problem-solving. Thinking is also slowed, but memory loss is not as noticeable as with Alzheimer's.

A brain-healthy diet is a vascular and heart-healthy diet, so if you have any hint of potential for stroke, you would do well to pay special attention to all the preventive tips in the Eight Weeks to a Better Brain program outlined beginning in chapter 11.

Lewy body dementia.[5] This is another common type of progressive dementia. It is characterized by abnormal clumps of alpha-synuclein protein, which has also been found in the brains of people with Alzheimer's and Parkinson's disease. Common signs and symptoms include hallucinations, acting out dreams in sleep, and problems with focus and attention. Other signs include the uncoordinated or slow movements, tremors, and rigidity that Parkinson's patients experience.

Frontotemporal dementia. This is a group of diseases characterized by the breakdown (degeneration) of nerve cells and their connections in the frontal and temporal lobes of the brain, the areas generally associated with personality, behavior, and language. This form of dementia manifests early – typically when people are in their 50s, and sometimes when they are as young as 45. It attacks the parts of the brain that control thinking, reasoning, and emotions. Common symptoms include radical changes in behavior, personality, judgment, language, and movement.

Mixed dementia. Autopsy studies of the brains of people 80 and older who had dementia indicate that many had a combination of several syndromes such as Alzheimer's disease, vascular dementia, and Lewy body dementia. There are studies going on now to determine how having mixed dementia affects symptoms and treatments.

Other Disorders Linked to Dementia

Huntington's disease. This is caused by a genetic mutation that causes certain nerve cells in the brain and spinal cord to waste away. This form of dementia is signaled by a severe decline in thinking skills, and it usually appears early in life at around age 30 or 40. Unfortunately, it is not readily eased by the Eight

Weeks to a Better Brain program in this book; however, using this program might help sufferers deal with some of the symptoms.

Traumatic brain injury (TBI). This condition is most often caused by repetitive head trauma. People such as boxers, football players, and soldiers might experience TBI.

Depending on the part of the brain that's injured, this condition can cause dementia symptoms such as depression, explosiveness, memory loss, and impaired speech. TBI can also cause parkinsonism; symptoms might not appear until years after the trauma.

The one positive aspect of brain injury resulting in dementia-like symptoms is that the brain is capable of compensating for such injury.

Symptoms to Watch Out For

If you lead a busy life with too much stress and not enough sleep, a questionable diet, and not enough exercise, you could have already set the stage for cognition problems in the future. As a result, you could begin to exhibit early signs of cognitive decline.

That doesn't mean that all is lost; it only means that now is the time to double-up on your efforts to improve your health so that you have the best chance of reversing any damage.

Review the symptoms below and see if any of them are presenting in your life or that of a loved one. Symptoms vary from person to person and with the type of dementia, but these are quite common:

- Memory loss: This is generally one of the first symptoms of dementia.
- Putting objects in odd places: Sure, we all set our keys down and forget where we put them. But if it becomes habitual, or, for example, you put them in places like the refrigerator, it can be a sign of something more serious.
- Difficulty learning and remembering new information
- Difficulty performing multistep tasks such as dressing or cooking; or in the case of cooking, forgetting that the stove is on or that you need to turn it on
- Problems going to sleep or staying asleep, especially if that has not been an issue in the past

- Changes in personality and behavior including agitation, anxiety, and aggression. This can also include becoming suspicious about family and friends.
- Confusion about dates, locations, and times for appointments, events, gatherings, etc.
- Having difficulty walking or wandering aimlessly or getting lost, especially in familiar places
- Repeating questions or having difficulty speaking or finding the right words
- Poor judgment or reasoning, which can also manifest as trouble managing money and paying bills
- Loss of sense of smell: One of the earliest signs of dementia is the loss or reduction of the sense of smell. The olfactory nerves directly connect to the brain from the back wall of the nose. If you cannot smell an open jar of peanut butter 10 inches from your face, you should get further testing.
- Trouble recognizing family and friends
- Difficulty reading, writing, and working with numbers

Unfortunately, many people who exhibit any of these symptoms avoid getting tested because they fear they will lose their job or their driver's license, or that they will be stigmatized. Please don't let that fear keep you from getting tested. There is a chance your symptoms indicate a serious medical condition other than dementia.

Sleep apnea, side effects of medications, depression, undiagnosed mental illness, and vitamin deficiencies can also result in such symptoms. And Lyme disease also mimics the symptoms of dementia. Recently it was revealed that actor Kris Kristofferson was misdiagnosed for years as having Alzheimer's when he in fact had Lyme disease,[6] so if you do get a diagnosis, make sure that you eliminate all the other possible reasons for the symptoms you're experiencing.

It is essential to know exactly what you're dealing with, so get tested.

Tests That Are Currently Readily Available

The standard tests offered by most physicians right now include a physical checkup including vital signs, bloodwork, and a review of your medical history. They also include cognitive tests including the Mini-Mental State Exam

(MMSE) and the Mini-Cog© test. Unfortunately, cognitive tests don't identify the true cause of many symptoms.

More reliable methods of diagnosis include positron emission tomography (PET) brain scans, which are expensive, and the analysis of cerebrospinal fluid (CSF) collected by a lumbar puncture. While these are more accurate, they are still not always definitive, so the hunt has been on to find more reliable, less invasive tests.

Tests That Look Promising

One test looks at fats in the bloodstream. It can distinguish between those who have dementia and those who are cognitively unimpaired, and between frontotemporal dementia, vascular dementia, and other conditions causing dementia-like symptoms.[7]

In a recent trial conducted by the National Institute on Aging, a blood test that looks for the brain protein insulin receptor substrate 1(IRS-1) showed that people with Alzheimer's had higher amounts of the inactive form of this protein, and lower amounts of the active form, than healthy adults.[8] The test is not widely available yet, but when it is released it will be able to diagnose early with a near 100 percent accuracy rate.

Measuring walking speed and hand strength is also showing promise as a predictor of the likelihood of developing Alzheimer's. Researchers at Boston University School of Medicine learned that individuals who had slow walking speeds and weak grip strength had a significantly higher risk of Alzheimer's disease.[9] These measures are simple, inexpensive, and easy to perform, and it is hoped that they will soon be used in any clinical setting to assess risk.

Another kind of blood test looks to be very promising. It measures the level of the Alzheimer's protein beta-amyloid in the blood and uses these figures to predict whether the protein has accumulated in the brain.[10] When this information is combined with two other major Alzheimer's risk factors – age and the presence of the APOE4 gene – it can predict with 94 percent accuracy brain changes in people with early Alzheimer's, even before there have been any symptoms. This test is still in trial stages, but hopefully it will be available soon.

In 2020, results of research on two other kinds of blood tests were revealed. In the first,[11] researchers measured levels of a protein called phosphorylated tau 181 (pTau181) and found they were able to distinguish people who had

Alzheimer's from those in a healthy group, as this protein presented as 3.5 times higher in those with Alzheimer's. In the second,[12] researchers tested blood levels of phosphorylated tau 217 (pTau217). They were able to identify individuals with Alzheimer's as efficiently as with the spinal fluid and PET scan tests. Unfortunately, neither of these blood tests will be available for widespread clinical use for at least five more years.

Retinal scanning also looks promising. The retina is made up of brain tissue and is connected to the brain via the optic nerve. Changes in the brain from dementia can show up in the retina.

In 2018, researchers at Washington University in St. Louis identified 30 people with no symptoms of Alzheimer's. They then did biological testing of these people for the plaques and proteins indicative of Alzheimer's disease. They used PET scans of the brain and examined spinal fluid. A little more than half of the subjects showed no signs of Alzheimer's in the biological tests. The others had the proteins or clusters of proteins found in the brains of people with Alzheimer's.

The researchers then used optical coherence tomographic angiography to scan the subjects' retinas. This scanning maps blood vessels in the retina. The scans of people who had biologic markers for Alzheimer's also showed changes in their retinas. In Alzheimer's disease the network of blood vessels thins and becomes less dense in the retinas.[13]

Other experimental diagnostic tests include a virtual-reality navigation test.[14]

The bottom line is that it is essential to know what you're up against, so don't hesitate to get tested. And if something does show up, you have even more reason to act now. You still have a lot to do, right? And you need your brain to do it.

Chapter 2

Understanding the Risks

I have a bit of good news and some not-so-good news.

First, the good news: Even if your parents or grandparents, brother or sister had or have Alzheimer's disease or another dementia, that does *not* mean you will get it.

Now the not-so-good news: Plenty of people develop Alzheimer's without having any family member with the disease.

That means there is something else at work here; and that something else is lifestyle. Information from many sources leads me to conclude that about 70 percent of cases of dementia can be avoided by making the right lifestyle choices. That means it's something for which you must take responsibility. But to do that, you need to understand the risks. And that's what we're doing in these next eight chapters.

Risk factors for dementia are also implicated in autoimmune diseases like multiple sclerosis and other forms of neurodegeneration like Parkinson's disease. Thus, by understanding them and doing what you can to control or eliminate them, you will have a much better chance of also protecting yourself from these and many other degenerative conditions throughout your life.

The conditions that set you up for dementia begin 20 to 30 years before any cognitive decline shows up. So even if you are only 30 years old right now, the mechanisms could have already been set in motion.

Even if you're a vegetarian or a vegan and have always worked out, there are other dangers that could be lurking from the past. Think about those amalgam fillings in your mouth. Or the asbestos insulation and lead paint that were in the house in which you grew up. Or how about the fluoride and other chemicals in the water you drink every day?

Some of us believe that living on four hours of sleep is a badge of honor. But you'll learn here that your insomnia is not just a nuisance when you're trying to concentrate. Lack of quality sleep can cause serious brain issues, so you must be more diligent about getting quality sleep every night.

In each of the next eight chapters is a series of questions that will help you analyze what risk factors are applicable to you. Consider these questions carefully, because they will help you evaluate your situation and prioritize the action steps you should take.

For example, if you already have an issue with inflammation, as with arthritis, chapter 3 is especially important. You will want to pay attention to everything that can contribute to that inflammation. Those swollen joints could easily have much more to do with your microbiome than with your calcium intake.

While many dementia programs deal mostly with your physical environment – food, exercise, toxins, sleep and the like, in *Don't Let the Memories Fade* you will learn how your mind and spirit also have huge impacts on your physical brain. We are what we think and feel, so the importance of good social interaction and a contemplative practice cannot be overstated.

Dr. Bruce Lipton reminds us that we are not at the mercy of our genes.[1] Whether or not "bad" genes get a chance to express themselves is largely due to our activities.

You have the power to save your brain now and prevent these terrible diseases in the future.

Chapter 3
Your Gut, Inflammation, and Dementia

Did you know that cognitive decline begins when we are in our 30s?

It's true that even though we may appear to be at our best mentally and physically, our brains are being impacted by the countless things that can cause brain cells to wither and die. We are all being exposed to external and internal stressors that can severely impact our brain health in the future.

The first is our diet, and how it affects our gut and our all-important microbiome.

I'll paraphrase here… "In the beginning was the soil, and the soil was good, and the soil had all the good things that man needed." Well, at least until the advent of chemical agriculture in the last century. In the past the soil did have all the nutrients that we and the plants that grew in it needed to thrive.

Soil has a microbiome just as we do. Unfortunately, the microbiome of most soil now is not healthy. Many of the beneficial microbes that used to thrive there have been killed by chemical fertilizers, fungicides, herbicides, pesticides, monoculture, heavy tillage, and the lack of organic matter they need to grow. (Think manure.)

Without soil microorganisms, nutrients can't get into or be utilized by the crops that are planted on the land. As a result, the plants are not only devoid of most nutrients, they are also unable to fight off insects and pathogens such as fungi. So farmers spray more herbicides and pesticides, and the soil becomes even more depleted. Then chemical fertilizers are dumped on the soil, which contaminates the groundwater and depletes the soil even further. It becomes a vicious cycle of spraying and fertilizing with chemicals until much of the soil is sterile and basically dead.

Many of the foods being grown in soil that lacks its original microbiome have also been genetically modified, because that's the only way they can endure that amount of poison. Corn, soy, alfalfa, and sugar beets are nearly all genetically modified now, and even zucchini, yellow squash, and papaya have been contaminated by genetic modification. Bottom line: the soil and the plants grown conventionally in it are sick.

Then there are the poor animals that are fed these crops. They are sick and stressed thanks to being raised in factories and being fed these genetically modified, pesticide- and herbicide-laden foods. They are raised in abysmal conditions, and are fed only to get fat, not in order to be healthy. They're also pumped full of antibiotics, which destroy their gut microbiomes. Those antibiotics become a part of the flesh and are passed on in the meat.

We end up ingesting plants and animals that are devoid of nutrition and filled with poisons from herbicides, insecticides, and who-knows-what-else. It's not difficult to imagine what that is doing to our bodies, particularly our own gut microbiomes.

Fun fact: Your gut contains 100,000 neurons. They are called the enteric nervous system. And your gut bacteria make over 30 neurotransmitters, including serotonin.

There are several microbiomes in each human: in the gut, in the lungs, on the skin, in the mouth, and there is even one in the female genital tract. All of them together are collectively "the microbiome," which refers to the entire collection of microbes in your body. More specifically it refers to the DNA of those microbes.

Why are microbes so important? A microbe is a tiny organism that is invisible to the eye, but it is the most abundant life form on Earth. Most microbes in your body are bacteria, but they can also be viruses and fungi. They are essential to your health.

An interesting study was done on mice. The researchers raised mice in a sealed environment, so they grew up with no microbial contact. As a result, their guts were leaky and did not develop properly. They also had compromised immune systems, weaker bones – and I have no idea how they measure this but apparently they were also depressed.[1]

We've been led to believe that everything must be sterile. God forbid you should let your kids play in the dirt outside or on a dirty floor. And with COVID-19, people were spraying and disinfecting shopping bags, door handles, and even the streets. All those disinfectants and chlorinated water eventually run off, and where do they go? Into the air, the surface water, and/or aquifers. These antiviral and antibacterial compounds that are everywhere in our environment are also helping destroy our microbiomes. And they can also have a huge impact on our mental health.

Destruction of the microbiome affects all the other systems of the body, including the digestive system, the immune system, the endocrine system, and even the neurotransmitter system. We'll start with the immune system.

The Immune System and the Brain

Amyloids is a general term for protein fragments that the body produces normally. In a healthy brain, amyloids are broken down and eliminated. But if the brain does not eliminate them, they clump together to form plaques that disrupt the signaling between neurons. These are the plaques found in the brains of those who have Alzheimer's.

Neurofibrillary tangles, which are also found in the brains of Alzheimer's patients, are insoluble, twisted fibers that consist primarily of a protein called tau, which forms part of a structure called a microtubule. The microtubule helps transport nutrients and other important substances from one part of a nerve cell to another. In Alzheimer's disease, however, the tau protein is abnormal and the microtubule structures collapse, so the nutrients don't get where they need to go.

One of the reasons most of the drugs developed so far to treat Alzheimer's have failed is that they are focused simply on removing or destroying these plaques and tangles. These drugs might do that for a while, but the structures always come back, often with a vengeance.

The reason? Beta-amyloid is an integral part of the brain's ancient immune system! Plaques form to protect the brain by encapsulating foreign invaders. One researcher called the plaques "brain pearls" that trap and sequester invading pathogens. Whoa! That means that when you destroy them, you encourage the brain to create more because you haven't addressed the reason they're there. Rather than destroying plaques and tangles, the answer to protecting our brains is to enhance and protect our immune systems.

And that's where the gut microbiome comes in, because the brain's immune system is intimately connected to the gut's immune system, which is intimately connected to the microbiome, the health of which is determined by lifestyle.

An unhealthy gut microbiome can lead to something called leaky gut,[2] which happens when intestinal components break through the barrier and into the bloodstream. The cells that make up the lining of the gut normally form tight junctions that allow through only nutrients such as amino acids, vitamins, and the simplest sugar molecules. But with a leaky gut these tight junctions weaken, allowing much larger, unwanted fragments to enter the bloodstream. This sets off an inflammatory response as the body tries to fight these foreign invaders.

A leaky gut also allows other bad guys like bacteria and yeast to enter the bloodstream. The immune system responds again, sometimes in a way that causes collateral damage to tissues, because to immune cells they resemble the invaders. In some cases this can lead to autoimmune diseases such as multiple sclerosis, rheumatoid arthritis, and lupus.

Another way your gut can be affected negatively is by parasites.[3] There are many kinds that not only affect the gut and immune system but also the central nervous system and the brain. It is difficult to test for parasites, but there are symptoms to watch out for, including constipation, pain in the stomach accompanied by mood changes and irritability, unexplained weight loss, and anemia. If there is any indication this is an issue for you, talk to an integrative health practitioner like a doctor of functional medicine or a naturopath. Parasites can even cause symptoms that mimic early signs of dementia, so it is important to be aware of their influence.

Inflammation in the gut from any of these causes is a HUGE contributor to dementia.

Poor Gut Health and Inflammation

There are two kinds of inflammation. One is beneficial. That's when your body responds to an injury like a cut or break or other wound and sends white blood cells, which destroy bacteria, to the site of the wound. This is a good thing; without those white blood cells jumping into action, a simple cut could kill you.

However, chronic inflammation, which keeps those white blood cells hopping, is bad for our brains. When inflammation is chronic, it stimulates production of, among other things, nitric oxide and cytokines.[4,5] This is a very simplified explanation, but basically these can increase the brain's production of the amyloid plaques and neurofibrillary tangles that cause Alzheimer's, because those are the brain's defense mechanisms.

In one report researchers aimed to determine if inflammation in midlife would have any consequences for the brain later in life, and they found there is a marked correlation between midlife elevation of inflammatory markers and reduction in the size of the hippocampus, the brain's memory center, as well as other parts of the brain.[6]

An unhealthy gut is a leaky gut, and if your gut is leaky, all manner of inflammation-creating substances can do their worst on your brain. Many people suffer from leaky gut and don't even know it, but your immune system and your brain know! Leaky gut equals inflammation, which equals danger to your brain. It can also cause damage to your heart.

What triggers inflammation? There are many factors, but we'll start with the most obvious: food.

Foods That Can Trigger Inflammation

1. **Trans Fats**

   Artificial trans fats are a primary source of inflammation. They're listed as "partially hydrogenated" oils in ingredients lists. French fries and other fried fast food, many margarines and vegetable shortening, and packaged cookies and pastries are sources.

   An imbalance in the diet between healthy omega-3 oils and vegetable oils' high omega-6 fatty acid content is also linked to inflammation. High omega-6 oils include soy and corn, and both of these oils are also often made from genetically modified crops, so they present a double risk for inflammation.

2. **Refined Carbohydrates and Sugar**

   Many studies link refined sugars, including high fructose corn syrup, to inflammation in the brain.[7] They also contribute to obesity and diabetes, which can lead to Alzheimer's (which I address in the next chapter).

   Remember when you are reading labels on processed foods, that there are at least 61 different names for sugar, including sucrose, dextrose, maltrose, and more. If you're not certain about an ingredient, visit one of the many online sites that list the various names used to hide this substance. I have also provided a link in the appendix under Week One.

   High-fiber, unprocessed carbohydrates are generally healthy if they are not from grains, but refined carbs raise your blood sugar level and promote inflammation. Besides turning into sugar in your body very quickly, refined carbs have also had most of their fiber removed.

Fiber feeds the beneficial bacteria in your gut; a lack of fiber can throw the ratio of good to bad gut bacteria out of whack, which leads to inflammation. Refined carbs can also increase the permeability of the intestines, leading to "leaky gut," which I discussed above.

While it's tempting to reduce your sugar intake by using artificial sweeteners, don't go that route. These sweet poisons have repeatedly been shown to change how our gut bacteria function, altering the balance and action of our microbes. They also mess with insulin receptivity, which comes up in chapter 4.

3. **Processed Meat**
Besides being associated with heart disease, diabetes, and stomach and colon cancer, processed meats contain more *advanced glycation end products* (AGEs) than most other meats. AGEs are harmful compounds that are formed when protein or fat combine with sugar in the bloodstream.

If you put the products that include them, like hot dogs, on the barbecue, you're looking at a prescription for inflammation, because cooking meats at high temperatures increases the amount of AGEs. This leads to problems with increased permeability of the colon, which means inflammation. Besides leading to brain issues later in life, this inflammatory response is also linked to the development of colon cancer.[8]

4. **Dairy Products and Meat from Factory Farms**
Grain-fed animals produce meat and dairy products that are high in inflammation-producing omega-6 fats. At the same time, they are deficient in the all-important brain-friendly omega-3 fats. These poor animals are fed mostly products that are genetically modified and drenched in pesticides, which are also connected to inflammation because they lead to leaky gut.

5. **Anything with Glyphosate**
Glyphosate damages the gut lining,[9] weakening the barriers that protect us on the inside from all the environmental toxins to which we are exposed. Anything that is not organic – wheat, most fruits and vegetables, and certainly anything from factory farms – contains glyphosate.

It can weaken the tight junctions between cells in the brain, which can result in a breakdown of the blood-brain barrier and lead to a host of neurological symptoms.

Remember those plaques and tangles that signal the presence of Alzheimer's? Your body constructs them to protect your brain. So if your brain is under attack from glyphosate or any other poisons, not only is there the potential for neurological damage thanks to the poisons, but the inflammation can cause your brain's protective mechanism to create more of those tangles.

Unfortunately, glyphosate isn't just in foods. It is poisoning the water and the air in most of the world. It has contaminated just about everything. It has been found in beer, wine, coffee, and many other products you would never think would contain it. Chances are you would test positive for it even if you eat mostly organic food from your own garden.

Other Inflammatory Triggers

Antibiotics

Antibiotics prescribed by your doctor don't just kill the bad bugs that cause infections, they also kill your good gut bacteria and thereby destroy the diversity of your microbiome.[10] Antibiotic residues are found in that factory-farmed hamburger you just had, the ice cream on your pie, and even the coffee you brew in the morning. All these antibiotics interfere with your microbiome's ability to do its job of regulating your metabolism, protecting you from toxins, and keeping inflammation in check.

Glyphosate is also actually an antibiotic. It doesn't just kill bugs in the fields, it kills the microbes and beneficial bacteria in your gut. So besides causing problems with inflammation, it makes you more susceptible to invaders like candida and Porphyromonas gingivalis (gingivalis).

Gum Disease

Recent research has linked gum disease (gingivalis, generally called gingivitis) to brain infection, amyloid production, tangles of tau protein, and neural damage in the regions and nerves normally affected by Alzheimer's.[11]

Researchers are not 100 percent certain how gingivalis gets into the brain, but there are a few plausible routes. Your mouth normally hosts a diverse but relatively stable community of bacteria. But when dental plaque builds up under the edges of your gums, it can form inflamed pockets in which gingivalis can thrive and release toxins. The inflammation and toxins caused by gingivalis[12] damage the lining of your mouth, which can make it possible for oral bacteria to enter the bloodstream and then other organs. Even if you don't have gum disease, transient damage to your mouth lining from eating or tooth-brushing can let mouth bacteria into your blood.

The blood-brain barrier should protect your brain from microbes, but gingivalis can invade white blood cells and the cells lining blood vessels, so it might cross the barrier via those cells. It can also enter your brain if your blood-brain barrier has been compromised; or it can invade cranial nerves near your mouth, then spread from cell to cell toward your brain over a period of years.

Candida

A recent study done at Baylor College of Medicine revealed that candida, which is a fungal infection caused by yeast, can easily cross the blood-brain barrier. The researchers found that once candida was in the brain, it triggered a massive inflammation response that quickly led to memory loss.[13]

The results prompted the researchers to consider the possibility that in some cases other fungi could be involved in the development of chronic neuro-degenerative disorders such as Alzheimer's, Parkinson's, and multiple sclerosis.

Hormones

Another thing to remember about the gut microbiome is that it is our largest endocrine gland. The gut has been called "the neglected endocrine organ." So even as an unbalanced microbiome can endanger the brain due to inflammation, it is also disrupting the hormones regulated by the gut. Those hormones in turn affect metabolism, behavior, appetite, growth, reproduction, immunity, and, of course, the brain.

When bad bacteria outnumber the good bacteria in your gut, your digestive tract is unable to eliminate excess hormones.

Time for a Checkup

Let's do a quick review and see how healthy your gut is.

1. How is your immune system? Do you find yourself succumbing to cold and/or flu viruses easily?
2. Do you deal with yeast infections often? This could signal a candida overload.
3. Do you suffer from gum disease/gingivitis?
4. Have you taken antibiotics in the last year?
5. Have you noticed digestive issues or any of the symptoms of leaky gut? Those symptoms can include food allergies, autoimmune diseases like celiac disease, rheumatoid arthritis, asthma, irritable bowel syndrome, excessive gas or bloating, and brain fog.
6. Do you have trouble losing weight even though you are sticking to a low-calorie diet and exercising?

If you answered yes to one or more of these questions, there's a good chance you're dealing with an unhappy gut microbiome.

And a question to consider if you suspect you have a parasitic infection:

7. Have you experienced or are you experiencing unexplained weight loss, constipation, or mood swings?

Action Steps

A well-balanced microbiome is essential for good gut health. If you have any inkling that your gut might not be working optimally, get a stool analysis. In addition to your family doctor, there are many online sources for this. That will help you know where you're starting from.

> *Important Note: If you're having severe stomach or digestive issues, you should be talking with your medical professional to get a full workup. If there is a practitioner of functional or integrative medicine in your area, I recommend starting there. You are a whole being, not just a stomach or a bowel.*

I provide a detailed dietary program in Eight Weeks to a Better Brain beginning in Chapter 11, but you can start right now by gradually adding some friendly bacteria to your diet.

Probiotics and Prebiotics

Adding fermented, probiotic foods like kimchee and sauerkraut to your diet is a great and gentle way to introduce good bacteria to your microbiome. Kefir water and kombucha tea are also beneficial. Yogurt is traditionally recommended as a source of probiotics, but dairy products cause inflammation, so go for plant-based yogurts like coconut or organic soy.

You'll need to give those good microbes some food, so also add plenty of wholesome prebiotics to your diet. Prebiotics are in fresh produce like Jerusalem artichokes, fresh dandelion greens, spinach, leeks, radicchio, frisee, endive, onions, asparagus, chicory, jicama, bananas, and garlic. There are lots of choices here, so no excuses.

In the chapter called "Foods to Eat, and Why" I provide a whole list of great foods, including fermented ones, that help build a happy gut microbiome.

Healthy Fats

Omega-3 fatty acids are essential to fighting inflammation. In fact, they are so effective that research has shown they can work just as well as anti-inflammatory drugs, without the side effects.[14]

Omega-3-rich plant-based foods include walnuts, flaxseeds, and hemp seeds. If you don't feel you're getting enough omega-3 in foods, you can take an omega-3 supplement, and there are excellent vegan versions.

Controlling inflammation is important for many other reasons besides protecting your microbiome. In chapter 4 we'll see how it has an impact on controlling diabetes and obesity.

Chapter 4

Diabetes and Obesity

You can have inflammation and poor gut health and not be obese. But if you are obese, it is likely that you also have poor gut health, which, as we saw in the previous chapter, contributes to inflammation and brain issues. However, this inflammation is not the only trait of obesity that increases dementia risk. Many people who are obese also have type 2 diabetes, and that is a serious risk factor for developing nearly all types of dementia.

Diabetes

In some circles, Alzheimer's is called "type 3 diabetes." That arises from the hypothesis that the disease is triggered by insulin resistance and insulin-like growth-factor dysfunction. This occurs when neurons in the brain become unable to respond to insulin, which is essential for basic tasks like memory and learning.

You might be thinking, "If that's true, am I doomed to develop Alzheimer's if I have diabetes?" The answer is no, but it is important to be aware of what could happen.

Over time, diabetes can throw off the balance of chemicals in your brain, which alone can trigger Alzheimer's. If untreated, diabetes can cause damage to the blood vessels, including those in your brain. Another factor connecting diabetes and Alzheimer's is that high blood sugar leads to inflammation.[1]

People who have type 2 diabetes might be up to 60 percent more likely to develop Alzheimer's disease or another type of dementia than people who do not have diabetes. And the higher the blood glucose, the greater the likelihood of developing dementia.

It is not just type 2 diabetes that is an issue. In the study noted in the Mayo Clinic article cited in footnote 1 above, middle-aged subjects with type 1 diabetes had higher rates of brain lesions and slower cognitive function than people without type 1 diabetes.

Severe hypoglycemic (low blood sugar) events are also problematic. If you experience an episode of extremely low blood sugar that requires medical attention, you have a two-fold increase in your risk of Alzheimer's disease.

And women should pay close attention. A study of more than 100,000 subjects who had dementia showed that, compared to people with no diabetes, after adjusting for possible confounders, women with diabetes had a 120 percent greater risk for the development of vascular dementia compared to a 70 percent greater risk in men.[2] Yikes!

There also seems to be a relationship between diabetes and Alzheimer's that could be tied to the Alzheimer's gene known as APOE4.[3] Protein clumps essentially disrupt the already weak insulin signal-processing, and this leads to starved brain cells. As a result, you have a higher risk of developing Alzheimer's if you have diabetes *and* have the gene.

If you have insulin resistance in middle age, you have a greater risk for Alzheimer's than someone younger with the same problem. It's thought this is because decreased brain glucose metabolism and dysfunctional brain insulin result in increased amyloid deposits and reduced brain volume.

If you then add obesity to this problem, you have the perfect storm for developing Alzheimer's.[4]

Obesity

A meta-data study (an analysis of many studies) showed that midlife obesity is associated with mild cognitive decline and Alzheimer's disease. In the referenced studies, it was found that obesity increased deficits in short-term memory, and that obese subjects also had deficits in executive function and increased rates of brain atrophy.[5] (Executive function is the cognitive processes important for reasoning, planning, and problem-solving.)

The good news, though, was that obese people who lost weight experienced low-grade improvements in cognition, attention, and executive function. This means that the cognitive deficits can be reversed to a limited extent.

A study published in the *Journal of the America Medical Association* (*JAMA*) showed that high body mass index (BMI) in midlife was the only midlife vascular risk factor that was significantly associated with more brain amyloid deposits in later life.[6] Other studies have shown that higher levels of all obesity measures were related to lower gray-matter volume.[7] Basically, the larger the belly, the smaller the memory centers in the brain.

Also, a higher BMI is associated with less activity in the prefrontal cortex.[8] This threatens our ability to make good decisions.

So consider this: If your prefrontal cortex is not operating correctly because of a high BMI, it is even more difficult to make good food and exercise choices, which can lead to more body fat, which can lead to more damage to the prefrontal cortex, which can lead to more bad choices. This vicious cycle could lead right to dementia.

This is corroborated in a study that found that participants who had a BMI of 25 or higher at the age of 50 were likely to develop Alzheimer's seven months sooner than participants who were at a healthy weight. And those who had a BMI of 30 at the age of 50 were likely to develop Alzheimer's an entire year earlier than those who had a BMI of 28.[9]

Other research has shown that fatty tissue itself secretes hormonal compounds that can contribute to dementia.[10]

With so many studies showing the impact that diabetes and obesity can have on brain health, you can see the importance of ensuring that you're doing all you can to get your weight and insulin sensitivity under control.

Time for a Checkup

1. Do you now have or have you in the past had issues with insulin sensitivity such as hypoglycemia or hyperglycemia?
2. Do you have diabetes?
3. Are you overweight?
4. Do you find yourself struggling to make the right choices with respect to diet and exercise?
5. Do you use artificial sweeteners like aspartame or sucralose?
6. Do you snack all day or have a snack before going to bed?

If you answered yes to any of these, now is the time to act.

Action Steps

The wonderful thing about the human body is that once you treat it right, it has an amazing ability to heal. If you are overweight or have type 2 diabetes, or both, a change in diet can likely solve those issues and protect your brain at the same time.

Removing sugars and refined carbohydrates from your diet is of course essential, but there are many other things you can do. Stay away from artificial sweeteners. Not only do they contribute to inflammation, they are also linked to obesity and increased risk for type 2 diabetes.[11] Drinks artificially sweetened with aspartame are found to triple the risk of stroke and dementia.[12] TRIPLE!

A new study released in March of 2020 found that sucralose, when combined with carbohydrates, makes it necessary for the body to release more insulin to achieve the same blood glucose level, an indication of decreased insulin sensitivity.[13] That can lead to metabolic dysfunction and weight gain.

A great deal of research is now emerging that shows that dairy and other animal products might have an even more detrimental impact on insulin receptivity than sugar! One example is with type 1 diabetes.[14] This is a disease resulting from destruction of the insulin-producing cells of the pancreas. Cow's milk appears to trigger the autoimmune response that destroys these cells, which then leads to diabetes mellitus in genetically susceptible people.[15]

That could be why people with type 1 diabetes who remove dairy products from their diet have found they do not need as much insulin. If you have type 1 diabetes, you might consider talking to your doctor about removing dairy products from your diet to balance insulin sensitivity as well as lower the autoimmune process, which creates the dreaded inflammation.

It's not just people who have type 1 diabetes who benefit from removing dairy products from their diet. Many of those who have type 2 diabetes have not only reversed their diabetes but lost substantial weight by doing so.[16]

Case Study: One of my clients, Irene, was having trouble managing her type 2 diabetes when she came to me, even though she was slowly losing weight and was eliminating processed carbohydrates and sugars. However, she was using yogurt, low-fat cheeses, and non-fat milk to get calcium, and her ankles and wrists were becoming swollen and inflamed. I recommended she switch to plant-based sources for protein and calcium. Within three weeks, her fasting glucose level was down to 80 and she no longer had the highs and lows she had been experiencing while consuming the dairy. She also had far less inflammation in her joints, so she was able to exercise more and consequently began to lose weight faster.

One interesting contradiction to popular wisdom regarding diabetes is with respect to fruit. Many healthcare professionals recommend that people who have diabetes or prediabetes should limit fruit consumption because of the fructose. However, fruit is dense in many nutrients, and increased fruit consumption has actually been associated with a lower risk of diabetes.[17]

⌘

It is far beyond the scope of this book to cover all the factors impacting diabetes, so I'm not going to get into all of them. I can, however, recommend checking out the Physicians Committee for Responsible Medicine webpage on diabetes,[18] a great article on insulin resistance at DrJockers.com,[19] and another at PlantBasedNews.com.[20] These resources will help you get a handle on diabetes, which is essential if you are going to save your brain.

For now, just start by removing dairy products and sugars from your diet, and moving toward a whole-foods, plant-based diet. You don't have to commit to a lifetime without cheese just yet. Try it for a few weeks. Give it three months. See how you feel.

Sleep is also essential to keeping diabetes and weight under control, so we'll deal with that in the next chapter.

Chapter 5

Sleep to Save Your Brain

In today's society, especially in North America, you often hear people boasting about how little sleep they need. It is a badge of honor to be able to function on four or five hours, for weeks on end. This is not something to be proud of. Sleep is as critical to your health as food and water. Poor sleep has been shown to increase your risk of Alzheimer's disease and other forms of dementia.

What happens when we don't sleep? Two specific hormones are affected when you don't sleep well. One is ghrelin. Lack of sleep leads to a 20 percent increase in the production of ghrelin, which is the hormone that makes you want to eat. Another one is leptin, which is the hormone that tells your brain "I'm full." When you are sleep-deprived, you have 15 percent less leptin.

Deep sleep regulates the growth hormone as well. Together with leptin and ghrelin, these three hormones regulate appetite. This means if you don't get enough sleep you'll want to eat more, especially sugar! Growth hormone helps turn fat into muscle. Increased muscle mass helps you burn calories more efficiently and improves insulin sensitivity. In other words, it stops sugar cravings and makes you thinner.

Lack of sleep can also elevate cortisol, the stress hormone. Cortisol is one of the most important hormones in the body and is released in a circadian rhythm. It is highest within 30 minutes of waking up in the morning and diminishes over the course of the day. But without enough sleep, cortisol doesn't regulate properly, leaving high levels that can poke holes in the gut. That can trigger disruption of the blood-brain barrier, which can trigger inflammation.

We also have something called the glymphatic system, which is responsible for removing waste from our brains. It acts just like the lymphatic system, which removes waste from our bodies. When we sleep, the glymphatic system gets to work removing toxins from the brain. But if we don't get seven to eight hours of sleep, the brain gets overloaded with toxins.

Another thing that happens when you sleep is that the proteins that cause Alzheimer's are actually "pulled out" of your brain, specifically during REM, stage three, and stage four sleep. If you don't go through all these stages of sleep, those proteins don't get pulled out of your brain, and this happens at the same time as other toxins are building up, cortisol levels are high, and your appetite is stimulated. In one study it was shown that just one night of sleep deprivation resulted in a beta-amyloid increase of 5 percent. That's one night! These plaques were found in brain regions including the hippocampus and the thalamus, the regions that are especially vulnerable to damage early in Alzheimer's disease.

While there can be substantial damage due to lack of sleep, there is also evidence that once you do begin to sleep better, some of that damage can be reversed. One study showed that cognitive decline was significantly reduced in Alzheimer's patients when they were treated for sleep apnea.[1] And another study found a reversal in cognitive decline in Alzheimer's patients who took melatonin to improve sleep.[2]

Sleep disturbances begin to occur years before the onset of Alzheimer's. If you have sleep issues, consider them an early warning system[3] alerting you to work on getting quality sleep.

Time for a Checkup

1. How many hours of sleep do you get per night on average?
2. Do you remember dreaming? Chances are, if you don't remember even snippets of dreams, you are not going through all the stages of sleep.
3. How long does it take you to get to sleep?
4. Are you able to sleep through the night?
5. Do you struggle to get out of bed in the morning, or do you jump up, ready and excited to begin your day?
6. Do you find yourself beginning to fade in the afternoon, or having difficulty getting through the day only to find you cannot sleep when finally you're able to put your head on the pillow?

If you are not sleeping well or it is taking you more than 15 minutes or so to go to sleep, it's important to figure out why and fix it… sooner rather than later.

Most of us use an electronic device just before going to bed. This includes watching TV, using cell phones, playing video games, using computers, and more. Many of us even sleep with cell phones nearby, with the ringer on. But the use of electronic screens and devices is negatively associated with solid sleep, and the more devices we use in a day, the more difficulty we are likely to have falling and staying asleep.

Diet is another factor. Deficiencies in nutrients like B_{12}, omega-3 fatty acids, and certain minerals are a recipe for sleep problems. And if you're like more than half of North Americans, you do not have sufficient vitamin D_3, which affects both sleep quantity and quality. A deficiency in this vitamin is linked to short sleep duration and a disrupted circadian rhythm. It can also result in a higher risk of sleep apnea.

Steps to Better Sleep

1. Turn off the electronic devices. The blue light from screens is disruptive to the production of melatonin, so you should stop using them at least an hour before bedtime. Turn off the wi-fi in your house before you go to bed. For many people, the electromagnetic frequencies can disrupt natural sleep rhythms, and in any event they are toxic, so it's better to shut off wi-fi whenever possible.
2. Create a consistent bedtime and waking-time schedule. Our bodies like regularity.
3. Make sure you have a well-balanced diet with adequate levels of vitamins D_3 and B_{12}, remove from your diet the inflammatory and high-glycemic foods (I will discuss the best foods in chapter 12), and make sure you have enough omega-3.
4. To ensure the best brain housekeeping is done while you are sleeping, eat your last food of the day at least four hours before going to bed.
5. Sleep in a cool, dark room. It's all about melatonin production, and melatonin is not produced well if you are too warm or there is too much light.
6. Create a sleep sanctuary. Keep it uncluttered and free of electronics and reminders of work. Think of it as your "Zen" space.
7. If you drink alcohol, do not do so within three hours of going to sleep.

8. For most people it's a good idea to stop consuming caffeine early in the afternoon.

9. Exercise every day, but no closer than four hours before bedtime. However, some people sleep well after doing specific gentle yoga poses before going to bed.

10. If you still have trouble sleeping, get checked for sleep apnea. It's much more common than you might think, and you must be able to breathe properly to get a good night's sleep.

11. Meditation is a great way to turn off your mind and enjoy a good night's sleep. Another wonderful tip is to make a gratitude list every night. As you're brushing your teeth or having a warm bath or shower, think about all the things you are grateful for that day. When you carry that with you to bed, you are carrying positivity to your slumber.

12. Take a warm bath or shower an hour or two before bed to relax the body and help with stress reduction.

13. Many doctors are now recommending cognitive behavioral therapy for insomnia.[4] This includes taking many of the actions I've mentioned above, and adds changing the thought patterns and behaviors that affect your ability to sleep or to sleep well. As you progress through this program, you'll see just how important positive thought patterns are for all aspects of brain health, so this is a highly recommended tool.

14. If you continue having difficulty, consider using some of the many natural supplements that help with sleep. Melatonin is one, and we're also now learning that it is neuroprotective. Valerian root, magnesium, passionflower, glycine, and lavender might also be useful for you. Just steer away from pharmaceuticals.

Sleep is controlled by the brain, and sleep controls the brain. Make it your friend, because good sleep is essential to saving your brain – just as important as exercise, which is up next.

Chapter 6

Move for a Happy Brain

Being sedentary is not just bad for your waistline, it is a serious threat to your overall health and disastrous for your brain. In fact, independent of all other risk factors, being sedentary gives you just as much of a chance of developing Alzheimer's as having the APOE4 gene. On the other hand, there is strong evidence that a lifelong habit of exercise can dramatically lower your future risk for dementia.

Many studies have shown that exercise can reduce Alzheimer's disease risk by up to 35 percent, and middle-aged women who are more physically fit can be up to 88 percent less likely to develop dementia.

When I say exercise, I don't mean that you have to run marathons or become a weightlifter. All you need to do is get your heart pumping, break a bit of a sweat, and get a bit breathless. You do, however, have to do it consistently.[1]

A 2019 study from Columbia University showed that any form of aerobic exercise, at any age, can help stave off age-related brain changes and enhance and improve cognitive function and cortical thickness.[2]

A 24-week study of 132 adults between the ages of 20 and 67 found that aerobic exercise increased executive function in adults as young as 20! What was fascinating from this study was the observation that the older you get, the stronger the effect of exercise, so that's good news for people who were not very active in the past.

These results are not just subjective. Brain imaging showed significant increases in the thickness of the cerebral cortex, independent of a person's age. This is especially important because the reason we lose some cognitive abilities during aging is that the cerebral cortex thins out as we get older.

A study from Germany showed a powerful connection between cardiorespiratory fitness and brain health.[3] Brain tissue is made up of gray matter, or cell bodies, and filaments called white matter that extend from the cells. The volume of gray matter correlates with various skills and cognitive abilities. The researchers found that increases in peak oxygen uptake during cardiorespiratory exercise contributed to improved brain health and decelerated the decline in gray matter.

For many people, the idea of working out in a gym is terrifying, so here's great news about aerobic exercise: It can be as simple as walking. That's right, walking is the easiest and best way to prevent dementia.

In one large study of almost 6,000 women researchers found that those with the highest amount of physical activity were less likely to experience cognitive decline during the six to eight years of follow-up than women with the lowest amount of physical activity. This study specifically studied walking as the physical activity.[4]

The leg strength you gain from walking is strongly linked to healthier brain aging[5] because stronger leg strength improves the flow of blood to the brain. One study of brisk walking showed that this increased blood flow to the brain leads to the release of a hormone called *brain-derived neurotrophic factor* (BDNF). This hormone helps stimulate the production of new brain cells and is attributed with making our brains "plastic," meaning they continue to grow and change. The presence of BDNF in petri dishes has caused brain cells to sprout new branches, which is essential for a cell to make new connections. If ever there was a reason to get out and exercise, this is it!

A hormone that was discovered a few years ago is called irisin.[6] It is released into circulation during physical activity, and researchers have found that it may promote neuronal growth in the brain's hippocampus, which is a region critical for learning and memory. There are also studies showing that physical activity can have an impact on brain volume as measured in an MRI. More physical activity, larger brain.

Another new and interesting study showed that workouts with different intensity provide different results for the brain. Researchers in this study discovered that low-intensity exercise triggers brain networks involved in cognition control and attention processing, while high-intensity exercise primarily activates networks involved in affective/emotion processing.[7]

This finding suggests that varying your exercise is a good idea. One idea to vary your fitness protocol is to add tai chi[8] or qigong.[9] They are excellent gentle exercises that increase strength and incorporate meditation with your workout. (You'll learn more about this in chapter 20.)

The benefits of exercise occur even if you've been mostly sedentary until now. A Columbia University study showed that the older a person was when they participated in aerobic exercise, the more pronounced the positive effect was on their cognitive function and cortical thickness![10]

Neuroplasticity

No doubt you've heard about neuroplasticity from TV ads and online, and you might be wondering if it's a real thing. It is. Our brains are "plastic," meaning they can grow and change. And exercise can help trigger neuroplasticity.

In a study published in the journal *Brain Plasticity* in 2020, it was confirmed that increased brain glucose metabolism and executive function followed 26 weeks of aerobic exercise training. Study participants who had enhanced physical activity as compared to those maintaining their usual physical activity showed cardiorespiratory and executive function improvement.[11]

Exercise also helps keep your weight in check. Since obesity is one of the primary contributors to dementia, adding some exercise to your weight loss plan can only help. Movement helps you burn more calories, and it helps brain function.

Time for a Checkup

Let's do a quick review and see where your activity level is.

1. Do you go for brisk walks every day?
2. Do you play any sports like tennis or do you swim or ride a bicycle regularly?
3. Do you do yoga, tai chi, or another gentle, meditative practice?
4. Do you do any kind of resistance training?
5. Do you go dancing or skating?
6. Do you play any team sports like soccer or volleyball or basketball?

The more of these to which you answered yes, the happier your brain is. If you do at least a half hour of aerobic exercise at least five days a week, you are well on your way to meeting the requirement for a healthy brain. If you also do resistance or weight training two or three times a week, you get extra stars.

If you're not doing much exercise now – change that.

Action Steps

Walk

If you're currently not exercising at all, just getting up and walking a block or two will make a big difference. Then add more blocks and more until you can go for 15 minutes or so. Then start speeding up to get your heart pumping.

Notice I said walking a block or two... not walking on a treadmill. Of course there will be times when you simply can't walk outside, like when there's a blizzard or it's dangerously hot, but do try to walk outside. Why? Because you also need vitamin D_3 and fresh air to save your brain. Get as much exercise as possible outside.

Add Some Music

Remember that you need to move fast enough to get that heart pumping and to feel a bit breathless. Sometimes it's hard to keep that up, or even to know if you're going fast enough. So keep up the speed by walking with music.[12] Brisk walking is 100 paces per minute. I like walking to anything that's disco... I never know when the mood may strike me to dance a bit while I'm at it. (Plus, it keeps the neighbors guessing.)

Which brings me to the next recommendation.

Dance

Dancing is amazing.[13] We'll be learning more about this in chapter 18, but it's one of the best exercises you can do. Our brains release endorphins when we dance.[14] These endorphins can trigger neurotransmitters that create feelings of comfort, relaxation, power, and fun. So not only do music and dance activate the motor circuits of our brains, they also activate the pleasure centers.[15]

And dancing is a social activity. As you'll see in chapter 18, spending quality time with others is also essential for keeping our brains healthy. With dancing, you can check off two of the most important things you can do to save your brain!

Besides the physical benefits, walking and dancing have been shown to protect against depression, which is a major contributor to Alzheimer's disease.[16,17] I'll be covering depression in much more depth in chapter 10, but know that every time you strap on those walking or dancing shoes and get out there moving, you're doing your brain a world of good from many points of view.

Do Weight Training

Strength and resistance training help cognitive function. At least one study showed that the amount of improvement that patients with mild cognitive impairment (MCI) enjoyed was dependent on how much strength they gained from the training. The stronger people became, the greater the benefit for their brains.[18]

This is good news for people who might have trouble getting out for brisk walks, because this kind of training can be done in the gym and easily modified for your fitness level.

Swim

An all-round excellent exercise, swimming is aerobic, it can include resistance training, and you can even get involved in exercise and spin classes in the water. If you have any kind of arthritis or joint pain, working out in the water ensures that you don't jar your joints.

&

Exercise is essential for good brain health. Do what makes you feel the best, but do it consistently. Aim for 150 minutes a week, combining aerobics and resistance training.

Chapter 7

The Toxic Brain

There are so many toxins in our environment, it sometimes seems overwhelming to even try to avoid them. They are everywhere – in your home, your office, your car. They're in the air you breathe, the water you drink, the food you eat, and even the clothes you wear.

But ignoring them doesn't make them go away, and the devastating effects they have on your body, your brain, and your mind demand that you be vigilant and do the best you can to mitigate the damage.

Let's start by examining some of the sources of these toxins.

Containers and Cookware

Bisphenol A (BPA)

BPA is one of the most common environmental toxins, found primarily in food and beverage containers. Ninety percent of U.S. residents have a detectable level of it in their urine, and studies have shown that the higher the urine concentration, the higher the risk for developing diabetes, a major risk factor for dementia.

BPA is also a known neuroendocrine disruptor,[1] which means it can mimic your natural hormones or bind to cells as your hormones do. As a result, your body believes there are higher levels of hormones than necessary, which can cause you to stop producing hormones or make your organs and glands work overtime to correct the issue.

Aluminum

You're exposed to aluminum in your antiperspirant, your cookware, and the foil around your baked potatoes. The link between aluminum intake and Alzheimer's and cognitive decline is proven, despite what the media wants you to believe. Aluminum is a neurotoxicant and promotes formation and accumulation of the proteins that are responsible for Alzheimer's.

A 2011 study published in the *Journal of Alzheimer's Disease* concluded that aluminum significantly contributes to Alzheimer's. The study author recommended that immediate steps should be taken to lessen human exposure to aluminum, which he said may be the single most aggravating and avoidable factor related to Alzheimer's.[2]

Another study released in 2014 concluded that Alzheimer's "is a human form of chronic aluminum neurotoxicity and ... chronic aluminum intake causes Alzheimer's disease."[3]

And if that isn't enough, a 2016 meta-analysis evaluating eight studies with a total of 10,567 participants revealed that people chronically exposed to aluminum were 71 percent more likely to develop Alzheimer's disease.

When you mix aluminum with fluoridated water, the dangers increase exponentially. Studies have shown that in the presence of fluoride (which is in most municipal systems in North America), aluminum leaches out of cookware directly into your food.[4]

Non-Stick Pots and Pans

Polytetrafluoroethylene (PTFE), known by the brand name Teflon, is one of the most toxic chemicals in your kitchen. Teflon releases at least six toxic gases when heated. One of them, monofluoroacetic acid, is known for being lethal even in small doses,[5] while another, perfluoroisobutylene (PFIB), is a chemical analog of the World War II nerve gas phosgene.

Perfluorooctanoic acid (PFOA) is another non-stick chemical used in the manufacture of Teflon. It has been linked to the development of tumors;[6] neonatal death; and toxic effects on the immune system, liver, and endocrine system. It is not metabolized by the body, so once it's in you (as it is in most humans living in industrialized nations) it's there forever.

Do not use this kind of non-stick cookware. Switch to a good quality stainless steel or safer non-stick. There are many safer brands of non-stick pans that use ceramic coatings, and new kinds are coming out all the time, so do research to choose the best available. Try also not to use aluminum pans or baking sheets in the oven; use oven-proof glass when at all possible.

The Air we Breathe

Air Pollution

Researchers of fine particulate matter say it has a direct effect on Alzheimer's disease,[7] and a report released in January of 2020 indicated that one's proximity to the pollution from roads is associated with a greater likelihood of developing all dementias, Parkinson's disease, and multiple sclerosis.[8]

Air pollution has been linked to the development of brain inflammation and accumulation of the proteins in the brain that are associated with Alzheimer's.[9] Depending on the kind of pollutants in the air, it can interfere with DNA synthesis, block the absorption of various nutrients, or destroy the bacteria that are so essential to gut health.

Toxic Scents and Sprays

Plug-in or battery-operated air fresheners utilize phthalates, which are also found in many plastics, aerosol sprays, paints, pesticides, cosmetics, and fragrances. Phthalates can cause allergic symptoms and asthma. Air fresheners also typically contain formaldehyde, which is a well-known human carcinogen that has been definitively linked to cancers of the nose and throat and irritation of the throat and airways, which can lead to dangerous infections, frequent nosebleeds, asthma, and other respiratory ailments.

Anything that interferes with respiration interferes with the brain, so don't use these products. In fact, stay away from any artificially created scents. Essential oils in a diffuser are much safer, and they have amazing medicinal qualities that we will be talking about in chapter 19.

Second-Hand Smoke

Second-hand smoke is fortunately not as big a problem as it used to be, but it can still affect people who live in homes where others smoke and those who work in bars, casinos, and the like.

Smoke from the lighted end of a cigarette, pipe, or cigar has higher concentrations of cancer-causing agents and is more toxic than mainstream smoke (the smoke a smoker inhales). It also has smaller particles, which can make their way into the lungs and the body's cells more easily. It affects the heart and blood vessels, which increases the risk of heart attack and stroke in non-smokers, and those are both risk factors for vascular dementia.

Do whatever you can to avoid it. And if you smoke – just stop. Seriously. Yesterday.

Toxic Sound

Research has shown that certain loud sounds, including from some music, can contribute to memory problems by damaging the actual hearing mechanism in two ways.

The first occurs when the sensory hair cells in your ears, which send neural messages, are destroyed by the sound. This can cause your inner ear to fill up with fluid which can ultimately lead to the death of neurons.

The second occurs when you have severe hearing loss. In this case, many traumatized neurons in the auditory cortex go dormant and don't respond to sound at all. Many remaining cortical neurons may still be able to react to sound, but in slow motion.[10]

Both these neuronal changes hamper your intellectual abilities, making it harder to engage in conversation and effectively communicate.[11] This can result in social isolation, which is known to make people more vulnerable to dementia.

Protect your hearing! If you must go to loud concerts, at the very least wear earplugs. When you're listening to music with headphones, keep the volume down. Avoid locales that have blaring music – it's just not worth the risk. If you work in a loud setting, be sure to wear proper protective equipment.

The Water We Drink

While we like to think of water in "first world" countries as being relatively safe, nothing could be further from the truth. Arsenic, lead, cyanide, acyclamide, mercury, chlordane, oxamyl, toulene, trichloroethylene, and bromate are regularly found in drinking water. Just as these chemicals cause cancers and other illnesses, they can also affect the brain over time.

Another area of concern with respect to water is that while aluminum on its own does not pass through the blood-brain barrier, studies have shown that when it is combined with certain compounds like those in fluoride, it can. Since many municipalities treat their water supply with aluminum sulfate and aluminum fluoride, the blood-brain barrier can be weakened, creating a pathway for aluminum and other harmful agents to get into the brain.

Speaking of air and water – the pesticides and herbicides used to grow our food don't just stay there on the plants or in the fields. They, too, are in the air and in the water.

Pesticides and Herbicides

Atrazine

Atrazine is the second-most widely used herbicide in the U.S. Like glyphosate and BPA, it is an endocrine disruptor. While other countries have banned it, atrazine is still used on North American crops and often winds up in the water supply. More than 70 million pounds of it are used annually to prevent weeds in fields, school yards, parks, playgrounds, athletic fields, and evergreen farms. Atrazine is often used with glyphosate on crops that have become resistant to glyphosate. Talk about a toxic double-whammy!

Glyphosate

Like atrazine and BPA, glyphosate is an endocrine disruptor,[12] which means it messes with your hormones. Your brain is deeply dependent on healthy hormone signaling for healthy functioning, so this is a huge concern.

A great deal of research has also shown that glyphosate destroys or dangerously alters the gut microbiota. As you've seen in chapter 3, an unhealthy microbiome means an unhappy brain.

The Body Toxic

Most of us do everything in our power to make our homes safe places, but they are in fact some of the most dangerous places for our brains. Especially the bathroom.[13]

Something you might find shocking is that the FDA permits arsenic, lead, and mercury in cosmetics.[14] Hair dyes, mouthwash, antiperspirants, deodorants, soaps, body scrubs, and shampoos all contain toxic chemicals, especially products that soap up a lot.

Toothpaste is also a problem thanks to the fluoride, sodium lauryl sulfate, and triclosan, and the food dyes in tooth gels. Aspartame and other artificial sweeteners add to the toxic soup.

Here is a list of additional dangerous chemicals in cosmetics:

1. Parabens are basically cheap preservatives that are hormone disruptors.
2. Fragrance… what exactly is in "fragrance" anyway? Could be any one of over 3,000 chemicals. Assume bad.
3. Phthalates are used to make products more liquid. You'll see them labelled as AKA, DPB, DEP, BBP, etc. They are connected to diabetes and ADHD, and thus are dangerous for the brain.
4. Hydroquinone, which is popular in skin-lightening products, has been linked to cancer, respiratory tract irritation, and eye damage.
5. Octinoxate, which can also show up as octyl methoxycinnamate (OMC) on the ingredients list, is a sunscreen chemical. But it is also found in hair color, shampoo, and some cosmetics. It has hormone-mimicking effects, is linked to inflammation, and is also suspected of contributing to cancer and thyroid problems.
6. Triclosan (an ingredient) and Microban (a brand name) are antibacterials that can and do destroy the good bacteria in your gut.

Isn't it interesting that better hygiene might be associated with increased Alzheimer's risk?! Countries like the U.S., Canada, and many in Europe including Sweden are considered among the cleanest countries in the world, yet they have extremely high rates of Alzheimer's.

When everything is sanitized, we are exposed to a far less diverse range of bacteria, viruses, and microorganisms, which means our immune systems develop poorly. This can lead to a myriad of problems including increased inflammation.

Just as you steer away from ingredients you can't pronounce in your food, do the same with personal care products. When you go shopping, remember that the term "natural" does not mean "safe" or "non-toxic."

Indoor Environments

In Our Furniture and on Our Floors and Walls

Common wisdom says that having flame-retardant materials in our drapes, mattresses, couches, and rugs keeps us safe. But nothing could be further from the truth. Every flame retardant is toxic and can cause serious long-term effects including cancer and digestive problems, which can of course contribute to dementia.

Lacquers can contain high levels of solvents that release volatile organic compounds, or VOCs, which can irritate eyes, skin, and lungs and cause headaches, nausea, and even liver and kidney damage.

Formaldehyde is in the pressed wood used to make furniture, and upholstery is often treated for stain and water resistance with a finish containing more formaldehyde and perfluorooctanoic acid. The fabric can be dyed with chemicals that are not adequately regulated but can cause allergic reactions in the short term, and brain damage in the long term.

This is a difficult thing to address, because every home has so many of these products in it.[15] If you feel you are suffering from toxicity, it would be wise to have your home analyzed by an expert in this area. Remove whatever you can that could be contributing to symptoms like brain fog, skin problems, and difficulty breathing.

Mold

A common contributor to Alzheimer's disease and other dementias is mold. Mold and other forms of fungus are dangerous microbes that can be inhaled from indoor environments that have hidden water damage. Mold can also exist in air conditioning and heating ductwork.

Researchers identified a subtype of Alzheimer's caused by these microbes inhaled through the nose, and labeled it *Inhalational Alzheimer's disease* (IAD). Researchers have found forms of mold and fungus in the brains of Alzheimer's patients.

Mold exposure can be treated, and this form of dementia has been reversed, although it is exceedingly difficult. If you have any reason, no matter how small, to suspect mold might be in your home or work environment, get yourself and your environment tested. Remove yourself from a mold-ridden environment right away so that you can be treated.

Heavy Metals

Heavy metals have been linked to the development of dementia in previous studies, but the relationship was cemented in a recent meta-analysis of a vast amount of scientific research.[16] The analysis revealed that there is a significant positive relationship between Alzheimer's risk and elevated serum levels of aluminum, cadmium, and mercury. As a result, the researchers strongly recommended that human exposure to these environmental toxic metals should be minimized.

Lead was associated with decreased risk for Alzheimer's in one study, but other studies have shown a relationship between an elevated lead level and metabolic dementia.[17] My thinking is it's better to be safe than sorry, and to avoid it.

The biggest danger from mercury is from fish and seafood, but many people also have it in their mouths in the form of amalgam fillings. The best way to eliminate this threat to your brain is to avoid eating fish; and, if you have amalgam fillings, get them safely removed as soon as you can.

Microwaves, Cell Phones, and Screens

As I am writing this book, there is passionate discussion about the dangers of the new 5G wireless system, but the toxic effects of cell phones and other wireless communication has been top-of-mind for many researchers for a long time.

It's far beyond the scope of this book to discuss the pros and cons of modern technology, but there have been studies indicating it can contribute to the risk for dementia. A U.K. study causally linked cell phone use to dementia. It was found that the damage was done through the creation of a leak in the blood-brain barrier.[18]

Another correlation was made in Germany. The location of the first microwaves/x-rays created on earth is near Frankfurt, Germany, so citizens living near the radio wave experiments were the first to be exposed to them. This is where Dr. Alois Alzheimer's first dementia patient was from.

A Chinese study concluded that the hippocampus can be injured by long-term microwave exposure, which might result in the impairment of cognitive function due to neurotransmitter disruption.[19]

Other studies have shown that when humans are exposed to electromagnetic frequencies of 50 to 60 hertz, there is an elevated incidence of Alzheimer's. Part of the reason for this is that these frequencies can cause an increase in calcium levels beyond that which is healthy. This in turn can lead to an increase in the production of Alzheimer's-inducing amyloid proteins.

There is also the danger of *digital dementia*, which is a term used to describe cognitive issues experienced by young people who spend too much time on phones and in front of screens.

These invisible toxins are difficult to avoid because microwave and cell phone radiation are everywhere, and with 5G being rolled out around the planet, it will be even more dangerous.

One way to protect yourself is to use cell phones only when necessary. The same holds true for wireless handsets for regular telephones. Turn off the wi-fi in your home when you sleep, and don't use microwave ovens.

Personal Interaction Is at Risk

Another big problem with electronic entertainment is that it tends to pull us away from human interaction. It is essential for brain health to have face-to-face contact with other humans. While this probably isn't a big issue for most people who are 60 or older in 2020, it could be a huge problem for people who are turning 60 in 2050. Social skills must be nurtured to make social interaction valuable for our brains. If a whole generation of people does not engage in quality, personal interaction with others, it could mean an even greater incidence of dementia in the future.

Headaches, skin disorders, mood disorders, allergic reactions like asthma, and autoimmune diseases are all typical symptoms of toxin exposure. Young people are experiencing memory issues as early as in their 20s. Brain fog, memory issues, and personality changes are also symptoms, and we can live for decades with these problems but never realize they are from toxic exposure. So let's do a quick checkup.

A Toxin Checkup

1. Do you have any kind of mysterious skin condition like rashes, dermatitis, eczema, or psoriasis?
2. Do you have frequent headaches?
3. Have you ever felt dizzy, had trouble breathing, or gotten a headache while using household cleaners or when you smelled gasoline or diesel fumes?
4. Have you become allergic to a food that you were always able to eat before?
5. Do you have or have you had unexplained flu-like symptoms that just don't go away? These can include any or all of fatigue, sore throat, upset stomach, fever, earache, and headache.
6. Do you have numbness or tingling in your extremities, or puffiness in your ankles, feet, legs, hand, wrists, or arms?
7. Do you often find yourself feeling overwhelmed or feeling like your brain is enveloped in a fog that you just can't get through? Are you getting forgetful?
8. Do you have trouble with infrequent or difficult bowel movements?

If you answered yes to more than one or two of these questions, your body might not be sufficiently flushing out the toxins you're exposed to. This is especially true if you live in an area with significant air pollution like that from factories, petrochemical production, or factory farms, or adjacent to busy roads. If you use common commercial household products, makeup, soaps, or toothpastes, you are being exposed to toxins on your skin and in the air in your home.

Action Steps

There is no way you are going to be able to avoid all toxins, but you can reduce your exposure by omitting things over which you do have control.

Around the house, don't use dangerous household cleaners, laundry detergents, and softeners. Baking soda, vinegar, and good old-fashioned water are incredibly efficient for most cleaning purposes. If you need to disinfect, use food grade (35 percent) hydrogen peroxide instead of bleach.

Be very careful with the food-grade product as it is extraordinarily strong. Dilute with water to 3 percent (3 parts hydrogen peroxide to 97 parts water). One small bottle lasts a couple of years. Store the 35 per cent mixture in the refrigerator.

On your body, switch to natural hair and body care products, toothpaste, etc. They are easy to find but be sure to read the labels carefully. Some toothpastes don't contain fluoride, but they still have the other dangerous ingredients like propylene glycerol, saccharin, and sodium benzoate, to name just a few. Again, good old-fashioned baking soda, coconut oil, or a 3 percent hydrogen peroxide solution work very well for cleaning teeth. And there are countless recipes online for other safe alternatives.

Food and Water

Organic food might seem expensive, but you can pay now, or you can pay later. Switch to organic food whenever possible. In the Eight Weeks to a Better Brain program you will eat a whole-foods, plant-based diet, so you're going to save money by not buying meat and dairy products. Spend those savings on quality organic produce.

Do whatever you can to avoid genetically modified foods. There are no studies showing these products are safe, or what genetic modifications can do to our brains, so it's better to just stay away from these foods. Remember that just because something is labelled non-GMO, that does not mean it's organic.

Assess the water you drink, shower, and bathe in. A water analysis can tell you how safe the water in your home is and whether or not there are elevated levels of lead, arsenic, and other chemicals or metals. Most places that sell filter systems can advise you in this regard.

Heavy Metals

Heavy metal toxicity is very serious. If you believe you are suffering from this, get thee to a specialist and get your blood levels checked. Then follow the protocol they recommend. This includes mercury from amalgam fillings. It is relatively easy to get these fillings removed, but you must go to someone who specializes in the procedure.

Turn Off the Screens Whenever Possible

Give your eyes and your brain a break – turn off your phone and tablet and computer and spend time outdoors in nature... ideally with real people.

Just because we live in toxic times in a poisoned world, it doesn't mean we have to let these poisons ruin our health. By being aware and vigilant we can protect our brains, and by reducing stress we can enhance our minds, so let's address this important risk factor next.

Chapter 8

Managing Stress Is Essential to Saving Your Brain

Stress is a killer. There is just no getting around it. If we still had posters up in post offices, stress would be up there as #1 Most Wanted.

When something happens, like an automobile accident, your body reacts with the stress response that has allowed our species to survive. It produces a brief surge of cortisol that gets you to move fast to get out of danger or gives you the strength to move someone or something out of danger.

Ideally, once you respond to the danger, cortisol returns to normal levels. The rush is over, and your body returns to homeostasis. For many of us, though, that stress response never gets turned off. Even though there isn't much that is truly life-threatening for most of us, our perceptions tell us otherwise.

We have been conditioned to stress about things that have no bearing whatsoever on our survival – things like unanswered emails and our kids not getting accepted to the best preschool. However, this perception of danger or urgency puts us into a state of continual stress. This leaves us exhausted, depleting our bodies of the energy needed to fight real invaders like cancers and viruses. The continual activation of the stress response results in a depleted immune system and a constant state of inflammation.[1]

This is because cortisol, the stress hormone, is immunosuppressive, and increases chemicals that suppress cytokines, which are the chemicals involved in regulating inflammation. As a result, the body and the nervous system and brain are in a state of chronic inflammation, which as we saw in chapter 3 is the root cause of many disorders.

Stress results in a lowering of melatonin levels, so sleep becomes difficult or impossible and, as we saw in chapter 5, that causes a whole raft of problems. Stress also contributes to depression, which itself is a risk factor for dementia.

You know those butterflies you feel in your stomach when you are getting ready to speak in public or to ask for a raise? That's a physical reaction by the flora and fauna in your gut. They are reacting to the stress, which weakens your microbiome.

Stress can also impact blood and oxygen flow to the stomach and weaken intestinal walls, allowing gut bacteria to enter your bloodstream, also leading to inflammation.

The constant presence of cortisol fuels the production of glucose, which is why stress is implicated in weight gain. Cortisol boosts energy to the large muscles but inhibits insulin production and slows metabolism.

Women handle cortisol differently than men do, and this is a big concern for us. For many women, high cortisol levels take down other hormones like insulin, thyroid, testosterone, dehydroepiandrosterone (DHEA), and progesterone, all necessary for a healthy gut and a healthy brain. This leads to anger, moodiness, and weight gain. This response to cortisol is considered one of the reasons women are twice as likely as men to develop dementia.

While the amount of cortisol produced in response to stress tends to go up with age for everyone, the bodies of women in their 60s and early 70s can produce up to three times as much as those of men in the same cohort. If your cortisol levels increase and remain high, it can have an adverse effect on the hippocampus, the seat of memory in the brain.

It's a Lifelong Thing

Stress has, of course, many sources. Traumatic childhoods, natural disasters, war, divorce, illness, financial difficulties – the list is endless. For many people stress is a way of life. They barely know any other state of being and they often don't realize what it's doing to them. But it's important to understand that stress is not just a one-way street. While external or perceived stress impacts the gut, stress can also *originate* from an unhealthy gut and/or a deficiency in essential nutrients.

Complicating this further, while nutritional deficiency can contribute to stress,[2] stress also increases your need for nutrients. The production of stress hormones and neurotransmitters uses many of your essential nutrients, but stress also shuts down your digestive system. That means that even though you are eating good food, and perhaps even taking supplements, they're not getting absorbed.

To save your brain, you really must get control of and deal mindfully and healthily with stress. So let's start with an inventory. What is your stress level?

Stress Test

1. Do you often get colds, the flu, or cold sores?
2. Do you often experience "butterflies" in your stomach just by thinking about something you must deal with?
3. Do you feel exhausted even if you've had a good night's sleep?
4. When you take a day off, do you feel guilty?
5. Do you find yourself getting angry and losing patience with people even over unimportant things?
6. Do you grit your teeth or sit with your shoulders hunched?
7. Does your heart sometimes feel like it's beating out of your chest, or do you have shortness of breath even though you haven't exerted yourself?
8. Do you often forget things?
9. Do you often experience indigestion, acid reflux (heartburn), stomach pain, nausea, diarrhea, bloating, or excess gas even after eating healthy meals?
10. Do your eyelids twitch?

If you answered yes to more than two of these, and they occur frequently, you probably need to address your stress level. It's easy to just say, "Avoid stressful situations, or don't let things bother you," but we all know that is much easier said than done. Many of us have literally no good stress-management techniques that we can call upon when we need them. The good news is…

Stress Management Is Not Rocket Science

There are countless stress-management techniques. When choosing one or more of them, pick something that works with your lifestyle and mindset. It doesn't matter what or how, just do whatever you've chosen consistently. Deal in a healthy way with your stress, or your brain *will* suffer.

I discuss more suggestions when we get to chapter 20, but below are some of the best and most common techniques. No, you don't have to go sit on a mountaintop and chant "Om" (although I hear that works well).

Most important, don't stress about your stress. Take it one step at a time, first by making sure your diet is healthy and promotes a healthy gut (see more in chapters 3 and 11), and then take however many of these steps you can. Do try meditation in some form, though, no matter what. It is incredible on many levels.

Meditation, Yoga, Qigong

By mindfully moving and holding postures in qigong or yoga, by chanting, and by breathing deeply and/or visualizing, our brains change. These simple processes can help prevent dementia because new neuronal connections can be formed and new neurons created.

Beyond that, these practices also help reduce stress hormones and inflammatory factors. While the protective factors are greater if you start these practices early in life, deep breathing and mindful movement are still effective even if you take them up at an advanced age.

Mild cognitive impairment (MCI) is one of the precursors of developing dementia. Symptoms of MCI include feeling overwhelmed, having trouble learning new things and staying organized, asking the same question several times, and having issues with communication. About half the people who suffer from it progress to full-on dementia. But a recent study found that a mere 15 minutes of daily meditation significantly slowed that progression.[3]

A study out of Los Angeles showed that participants who practiced yoga and meditation had more improvements in visual-spatial memory skills – the ability to navigate and remember locations – than participants who engaged in memory-enhancement training. The yoga and meditation group members also scored better on stress resilience and had lower levels of anxiety and depression.[4]

This does not take hours and hours a day – it can be as little as 15 minutes a day. What do you have to lose besides stress?

You don't have to spend a lot of money, either. There are many great online programs and free YouTube videos to help you begin these practices. A few of them are referenced in the appendix.

Exercise

We know that exercise is good for the brain (chapter 6) but with respect to stress management, think endorphins – the feel-good hormones. Even the Mayo Clinic recommends exercise for stress reduction.[5]

Listen To or Make Music

Nothing calms me down better or faster than playing my harp. Most people obviously don't have this particular luxury, but you probably have access to some kind of instrument. A piano, a guitar, a drum – heck, even a recorder will do. And we all have access to our voice, the original instrument. Studies have shown that singing reduces stress, and even more so when singing in a group. It releases endorphins and oxytocin, a hormone that lowers stress and creates bonding.

Making music is an awesome stress reliever provided you don't start stressing about how well you're doing it. Just enjoy the process of playing or singing. Don't worry about the results. Bonus side effect: The very act of playing music improves the structure of your brain. More on that in chapter 18.

Listening to music that is pleasing to you physiologically lowers the production of stress hormones[6] and increases dopamine production.[7] I personally like light classical or ambient music, but if good old rock 'n roll or jazz helps you chill, that's the music for you.

Stress-Busting Supplements

I'm prefacing this section by saying that I am not an herbalist, Ayurvedic practitioner, or doctor. I'm a vegan nutritionist and a researcher into brain health. I cannot "prescribe" anything, and I highly encourage you to check with your doctor or integrative practitioner if you decide to use supplements to help reduce stress.

Among the best are gamma-aminobutyric acid (GABA), lemon balm, and ashwagandha. The neurotransmitter GABA can induce relaxation, analgesia, and sleep, so it directly affects your personality and your capability to manage stress.[8] You need at least 250 mg two or three times throughout the day. Some experts recommend taking it all the time, but many also say it's fine to just take it when you're feeling stressed or anxious.

Lemon balm is useful for a couple of reasons. First, it can effectively increase GABA activity in the brain. Second, it inspires activity at specific brain receptors to help them respond to the neurotransmitter acetylcholine, which is integral to logical thinking, formation of memories, basic cognition skills, and working memory capacity.[9] How much? Three hundred to 500 mg per day – but always try for as low a dose as possible. Lemon balm is also available in tea form, so this might be a great way to incorporate it into your regime.

Ashwagandha is another powerful herb that has been used for centuries in Ayurvedic medicine.[10] It can lower your cortisol levels by 28 percent and it promotes restorative sleep. It has so many uses that it's a staple for many who are into alternative health methodologies. Take one or two teaspoons (3 to 6 grams) of dried ashwagandha root powder per day. *Do NOT take this if you are pregnant.*

Other stress-reducing nutrients include magnesium, calcium, the B vitamins, vitamin D_3, zinc, and tryptophan.

Get Outside

One of the best ways to reduce stress *and* build up the immune system is to get outside in nature, and even more important, to exercise in nature. There has been a great deal of research on this topic; one of the most notable studies came from New Zealand where it was found that even just a view of a body of water helped significantly reduce stress.[11]

You might not be able to go on a retreat in the country, but you can get outside in a park, by a river, or near the ocean. Do whatever it takes because it *will* help you deal with stress in a healthy way.

༄

Just as getting enough and the right kind of sleep is essential to saving your brain, getting stress under control is not an option. Nor is having healthy social interactions, the topic of the next chapter.

Chapter 9

Alone or Lonely? Your Brain Knows

To me there is nothing sadder than seeing an elderly person sitting alone at a window, looking out at the world day after day, with no visitors, no meaningful social interaction, no conversation.

We had a neighbor whose mind was very sharp, even to the age of 92. He was a social butterfly and was always out and about. But when his lungs began to fail and he could no longer get out and walk around or drive to the store or join his morning coffee group, his mental decline was staggeringly fast. Even though neighbors would stop in to visit and bring treats, the isolation really got to him, and it was within only a few months that the light went out in his eyes and he began the inexorable slide into dementia.

My mom was a brilliant businesswoman and was a master of conversation when it came to her passion, which was dolls. But after she retired and closed her store, she quickly began to decline mentally. When her ability to remember words began to diminish, she pulled away from others, even friends who shared her passion. She was embarrassed because she could not convey her thoughts. She stopped going out to visit and even began to refuse letting others come to visit her.

Her social circle soon consisted only of my sister, my sister's husband, my dad, and myself. We could not convince her to spend any time with others, and so she lost her ability to communicate very rapidly.

What happened to our neighbor and to my mom is very typical of what happens to people who suffer from chronic social isolation, and I'm hoping their stories inspire you to pay close attention to the importance of quality time with others.

The Dangers of Social Isolation

Research suggests that isolation can cause an overproduction of a neural chemical that can make mammals more fearful and aggressive, which can increase stress, which of course increases the likelihood of developing dementia.[1]

Social isolation is also dangerous for people who are already experiencing stress. Without interaction, they do not have the coping mechanisms they need, which further exacerbates the effects of stress on the body and the brain.

The connection between isolation and depression in humans, and between feelings of loneliness and depression, especially among the elderly, is well established.[2,3] Isolation-induced depression can and often does manifest as dementia.[4]

Long-term social isolation is linked to an increased risk of premature death. In fact, Dr. Julianne Holt-Lunstad, a professor of psychology at Brigham Young University, analyzed 70 studies that included more than 3.4 million participants, and concluded that loneliness, social isolation, and living alone were more of a threat to a person's health than obesity.[5]

Chronic isolation has been linked to chronic inflammation as well, and of course inflammation is intimately involved in the development of dementias of all kinds.

Loneliness, even if a person is among other people but feels lonely, is significantly associated with impaired psychomotor processing speed and delayed visual memory,[6] both symptoms and precursors of dementia.

We are social animals. We need to spend time with others. Unfortunately, an increasing portion of the world's population experiences isolation regularly, thanks in part to families spread far apart. The technology that keeps people glued to screens instead of spending personal time with each other is also dangerous. And now, in 2020, is the incredibly dangerous mandate that people be isolated due to the COVID-19 virus. I believe that we will see increased instances of cognitive decline, and certainly mental health issues, as a result.

Checkup: What's Your Level of Social Interaction?

1. Do you spend quality time with a significant other or good friends?
2. Do you participate in clubs or groups or do you volunteer?
3. Do you have a healthy relationship with your children/spouse/parents?

4. Do you go dancing or sing in a group or attend a church or other religious institution?
5. Do you participate in exercise or swimming or yoga classes?
6. Do you enjoy your time alone, or do you struggle with feelings of loneliness?

Be honest, and if you're not spending quality time with others, consider why that is. Are you having hearing problems? Are you physically challenged? Try not to let the status quo put you at risk for brain issues later. Reach out!

The Value of Quality Social Interaction

Many studies have shown that a good social network is directly correlated to a decreased risk of developing Alzheimer's and a slower rate of cognitive decline. One six-year study involved 593 participants over the age of 65 who were free of dementia at the beginning of the study. The participants' social interactions were monitored, as were their cognitive abilities. Those with higher levels of social interaction, which included activities like traveling, having an active approach to life, and maintaining an active social life, were less likely to develop dementia.

Another study revealed in the *Journal of Alzheimer's Disease* involved people who did not have dementia who participated in a highly interactive discussion group while others in the study participated in tai chi, walking, or were part of a control group who received no interventions. Those involved in the discussion group not only improved their cognitive function, but MRIs showed that their brain volumes also increased.

For people who are already showing symptoms of MCI, research has demonstrated a decreased risk of progression to dementia for those who actively participate in social activities such as volunteering, going to a place of worship, attending special family occasions, going to restaurants, and attending organizational activities.

Researchers have also explored the effect of neighborhood[7] and midlife marital status[8] on the risk of developing dementia. Healthy social bonds with peers or a marital partner appear to lend a beneficial effect on cognition in older age.

Action Steps

There are many things you can do to improve your level of social interaction. This is especially true if you are retired or even if you are a caregiver. It's important to make contact with people outside your home.

Volunteer to read to kids at a library or help out in your grandkids' classroom. Spend time at a nursing home and play games or just chat with the residents. Join a religious group or audit classes at a local college.

Sometimes problems with hearing or seeing can make it difficult to get out, so if you need glasses or hearing aids, get them and use them. (See more about this in chapter 10.)

&

Making the effort now to experience new adventures and participate in favorite activities with people who enhance your life can make a huge difference to your physical and mental health going forward. Enjoy the company of others now, for a healthier and more vibrant future with many wonderful memories.

Chapter 10

Miscellaneous Threats to Your Brain

This is the final chapter in the "Challenges" section, but being last is definitely not least. Here you'll learn how depression, hearing loss, heart disease, smoking, and other triggers can threaten your cognitive health.

Depression

Depression is one of the most common conditions affecting older adults, estimated at about 15 percent of people over age 65. Persistent feelings of sadness, lack of energy, memory disturbances, loss of interest in things that would normally give them joy, and changes in normal eating and sleeping are some of the symptoms.

Wait a minute… what do those symptoms sound like? You guessed it: early dementia. This is one of the many reasons it's essential to understand that many conditions can mimic dementia, so it's important to have the diagnostic tests to determine what is actually going on.

Depression is a common antecedent of Alzheimer's. Researchers in one study found that depressed older adults (defined as those over age 50) were more than twice as likely to develop vascular dementia and 65 percent more likely to develop Alzheimer's disease than similarly aged people who weren't depressed.[1]

But it's not just late-life depression that is related to the risk. A history of depression in younger years can double the risk of developing Alzheimer's.

The author of a 2011 paper estimated that almost 15 percent of Alzheimer's disease cases in the United States are "potentially attributable to depression."

He further surmised that a 10 percent reduction in depression might prevent 68,000 cases of dementia. That's just in the U.S.[2]

What's the Connection?

We're not 100 percent clear about the causal relationship between depression and dementia. One possibility is inflammation of brain tissue. Some evidence links chronic low-grade inflammation with changes in brain structure.[3] For example, neuronal loss is common in major depression. The progression from depression to dementia could happen as a result of the activation of macrophages in the blood and microglia in the brain that release proinflammatory cytokines. These could lead to the neurodegenerative changes associated with Alzheimer's disease and other dementias.

Certain proteins increase in the brain with depression, and they might also increase the risk of developing dementia. Additionally, the stress hormones created when one is depressed can contribute to brain shrinkage and dementia. (See chapter 8.)

Low magnesium levels have also been tied to increased rates of depression,[4] just as they have with dementia. And another important factor that we know contributes to both depression and dementia is an unhealthy gut.

Dietary changes have proven to be an excellent way to treat depression and help prevent dementia. A study from the University of Michigan found that when patients ate a diet designed to ease digestive issues, they reported an increased sense of quality of life and decreased anxiety and depression.[5] In another trial, researchers found that a healthy diet had a powerful impact on depression. Depressed patients were treated with diet or social support. Compared to those with social support, those with the healthy diet tended to stay in the study longer and many found their depression going into remission.[6]

Action Steps for Depression

If you suffer from depression, it is essential that you deal with it. Depression makes it much less likely that you will follow a healthy lifestyle. It saps your energy and motivation, so the very lifestyle factors that protect you from dementia, like diet and exercise and social interaction, are disrupted.

If you're not already working with an integrative practitioner, find one to help you get better nutrition and more exercise and confront and deal with negative thoughts. In the meantime, get started looking after your gut. Remove processed foods, sugars, and wheat products from your diet, and make sure your vitamin B$_{12}$, folic acid, and magnesium levels are in the healthy range. (See chapter 15.)

Remove unhealthy fats from your diet. When participants in a large study replaced less healthy vegetable oils with olive oil, their risk of depression plummeted by almost 50 percent.[7]

The essential fatty acids docosahexaenoic acid (DHA) and eicosapentaenoic acid (EPA) can help because these fats support serotonin – a nerve messenger that helps balance your mood. They also have anti-inflammatory effects on nerve cells, reducing further the possibility of developing dementia.

Cognitive behavioral therapy has been shown to help mild to moderate depression.[8] A trained therapist in this modality can help you identify false or negative thoughts and replace those thoughts with healthier, more realistic ones.

Meditation is also enormously powerful.[9] It is a proven therapy with no dangerous side effects! There is a lot more about meditation in chapter 20.

Pharmaceuticals

A meta-analysis of dozens of studies showed that antidepressants do not work in most cases of depression,[10] especially when depression is a result of inflammation.[11] And while they are often not effective for their prescribed use, like many other pharmaceuticals they do have an enormous negative impact on the health of the brain.

People who have taken a type of drug called anticholinergics, which can be found in sleep aids and allergy medications, are more likely to develop dementia.[12] This is largely because these medications can lower the level of the brain chemical acetylcholine, which is an important messenger in memory pathways. This is true even if the drug was used 20 years ago.

Another class of drugs that has been linked to dementia is proton pump inhibitors. According to a study in *JAMA*, dementia was 44 percent more common in those on acid-blocking drugs. Why? A study released in May of 2020 explained that these drugs lead to degeneration of neuronal networks, which can lead to cognitive impairment and movement disorders.[13] If you're using proton pump inhibitors, check your diet. If you need acid reduction, that is probably because your gut is unhealthy. Stop eating processed junk food and address the health of your gut.

Long-term use of benzodiazepines (you may know them as Valium or Xanax), which are frequently prescribed for anxiety and sleep problems, appears to be linked to an increased risk of developing Alzheimer's disease.[14] These same drugs can also increase the risk of an earlier death for those with dementia. This is so serious that the U.S. FDA now mandates that drug makers add what is referred to as a "black box" warning to the labels of all antipsychotics, alerting doctors and patients to this increased mortality risk in people with dementia-related psychosis. If you take benzodiazepines, have you considered that your anxiety might be related to your gut health? (See chapter 3.) If you are on this medication, a serious discussion with your doctor is in order.

Another drug, oxybutynin, which is prescribed for overactive bladder in elderly patients, has been linked to thinking problems and increased risk of dementia in older people.[15]

Anti-inflammatories and painkillers are also connected to serious gut issues, and rather than getting rid of the source of the inflammation, they simply mask the problem. Analyze your issues. If you have back or knee pain, would yoga or weight loss help? If you have headaches, diet and stress have an enormous influence. By improving your diet and dealing with the stress, you should be able to eliminate the painkillers or anti-inflammatories. Systemic inflammation not only causes pain, but it affects your brain. So rather than taking a drug to mask it, figure out where the inflammation is coming from. Does drinking a beer make your joints hurt? Does having toast make your hands swell? By analyzing what triggers your pain or inflammation, you can remove that from your diet and eliminate the need for the medications.

Action Steps

Work with your general practitioner or an integrative practitioner to reevaluate why you are on any medications, and shift to dealing with the root problem if possible instead of endangering your brain with pharmaceuticals.

Surgeries

Left-heart catheterization is one common procedure that has a proven connection to MCI. Eight to 13 percent of patients who have the surgery have been found to have MCI three months after the procedure.[16]

Mayo Clinic research linked exposure to general anesthesia to a subtle decline in memory and thinking skills in adults over 70.[17] Although the decline in brain function was small in most cases, this could be a serious problem for anyone who is already suffering from cognitive decline. And if an older adult has borderline cognitive functions that have not become obvious yet, exposure to anesthesia and surgery could unmask problems with memory and thinking.

Action Step

If you are considering having surgery that involves general anesthesia, it would be a good idea to discuss the likelihood of future problems with your surgeon and your anesthetist. If it is elective surgery, you may want to reconsider.

Smoking

Not everyone who smokes will get dementia, but a World Health Organization study showed that smokers have a 45 percent higher risk of developing dementia than non-smokers.[18] Smoking was also one of the nine modifiable risk factors highlighted in the 2017 Lancet Commission on dementia risk.[19] There is such a strong relationship between smoking and dementia that some researchers estimate that 14 percent of dementia cases worldwide might be attributable to smoking.[20]

The two most common forms of dementia, Alzheimer's and vascular dementia, have both been linked to problems with the vascular system (heart and blood vessels). Smoking increases the risk of vascular problems, including via strokes or smaller bleeds in the brain, which are also risk factors for dementia. In addition, toxins in cigarette smoke increase oxidative stress and inflammation, which have both been linked to developing Alzheimer's disease.

The good news is that when you stop smoking, there is a reduction in your risk of dementia.

Second-hand smoke is also dangerous. Not only has it been shown to increase the risk of cancer, cardiovascular disease, and other diseases, several studies have suggested that the same holds true for dementia.[21]

Action Step: Stop. Just Stop. Do. Not. Smoke.

Alcohol Consumption

According to most studies, it appears that excessive alcohol consumption over a lengthy time can lead to brain damage[22] and might increase the risk of developing dementia.

The brain's white matter, which helps transmit signals between different regions of the brain, is more likely to be reduced in heavy drinkers. This affects how the brain is functioning. Heavy drinking can also cause vitamin B₁ (thiamin) deficiency and Korsakoff's syndrome, which is a short-term memory disorder.

On the other hand, moderate consumption has not been conclusively linked to an increased dementia risk, and at least one meta-study[23] seemed to indicate that moderate alcohol consumption might offer some protection against developing dementia. A maximum of one drink daily for women and two drinks daily for men is considered moderate drinking.

Action Step

Save your alcohol consumption for a special event like a birthday or have an occasional glass of wine.

Hearing Loss

Many studies have shown an association between cognitive decline and hearing loss, and that hearing loss can contribute to cardiovascular disease, depression,[24] and the risk of falls,[25] all of which are linked to an increased risk of developing dementia.[26]

A project at Johns Hopkins followed 2,000 seniors over six years, looking at a possible relationship between cognitive decline and hearing loss. All the volunteers were cognitively normal at the beginning of the study, but by the end, people with hearing loss were 24 percent more likely to meet the criteria for a diagnosis of cognitive decline than were those with normal hearing.[27]

Memory can also be adversely affected by hearing loss. If you can't hear information clearly, the brain's ability to remember it is diminished. Hearing loss can also mean that the brain is not being adequately stimulated,[28] which leads to cognitive decline.

How's Your Hearing?

If you show any of the following symptoms, take the time and make the effort to get your hearing checked.[29]

- Speech or other sounds seem muffled
- Difficulty understanding words, especially if there is background noise or you are in a crowd
- Trouble hearing consonants
- Frequently asking others to speak more slowly, clearly, and loudly
- Needing to turn up the volume of the television or radio
- Withdrawal from conversations
- Avoidance of social settings where hearing is an issue

Action Steps

If you do not have hearing loss, do your best to prevent it in the future. Hearing loss can happen from continuous or frequent exposure to loud noises, a head injury, a stroke, or even intense pressure as in scuba diving.

Wear sound-cancelling over-the-ear headphones if you work in loud environments. Protect your ears at all costs from shocks.

Ear infections can easily cause hearing loss, so have them treated promptly.

If you are suffering hearing loss, don't ignore it. Many people don't want to accept that their hearing may be compromised. My dad was in that group, and it was a struggle to get him to wear his hearing aids. But showing him how hearing loss can contribute to dementia convinced him that the inconvenience is far less than that of losing his mind!

No doubt hearing aids can be expensive, but there are other options currently showing up in the marketplace, like sound-amplification devices sold at places like Amazon.[30,31]

Vision Loss

Data from two large studies showed that older people who have problems with distance vision (worse than 20/40) are two to three times as likely as those with strong vision to be cognitively impaired. Even the perception of having bothersome vision problems was associated with higher odds of cognitive impairment.[32]

In another study of 1,061 women, researchers found that, compared to their peers with good vision, the women with visual problems were at two to five times the risk of having dementia or MCI. Memory problems were most pronounced in women whose vision was worse than 20/100 on eye exams.[33]

Like poor hearing, poor vision is a form of sensory deprivation, so the brain is getting limited stimulation. Vision impairment can also lead to social disengagement.

Action Steps

Eye diseases like macular degeneration, diabetic retinopathy, and glaucoma are common in elderly people. It's important to get your eyes tested. If you need glasses, wear them. If cataract surgery is indicated, which generally only requires a local anesthesia, just do it.

Poor Posture

Poor posture doesn't just cause pain and degeneration in the muscles and skeletal system, it also negatively impacts the brain. The spine is the motor that drives the brain, and if it isn't aligned, neither is your brain.

According to the research of Nobel Prize recipient Dr. Roger Sperry, 90 percent of the stimulation and nutrition to the brain is generated by the movement of the spine.

But we have a big problem these days: the phone slouch. People are leaning over their phones or tablets for hours every day, developing what has been called "forward head posture." Their spines are curved completely out of line, and they remain in that position for hours.

This is bad for a few reasons. Every time we lean forward 60 degrees, the stress on our necks is increased by approximately 60 pounds. As a result, forward head posture leads to chronic pain, numbness in the arms and hands, improper breathing, and pinched nerves.

That's just the beginning. That posture puts undue strain on our necks and spinal cords, which has a negative impact on feelings of stress, mood, memory, and even behavior. Slouching also affects the position and function of your abdominal organs, inhibits breathing and oxygen intake, and causes headaches.

A low oxygen level, depression, and digestive problems are all contributors to the likelihood of developing dementia, so it's important to be aware of and correct your posture now.

According to Harvard Health, "Good posture means keeping the cervical, thoracic, and lumbar curves in balance and aligned, with weight distributed evenly over the feet."[34]

Check Your Posture

Check your posture and your neck alignment. One way is to stand against a wall with your heels, pelvis, upper back, and head all touching the wall. Keep your chin parallel to the floor. This should be easy and comfortable.

Then, staying in place, slide your hand between the wall and your lower back. Keep your chin parallel to the floor. If you can't get your hand in past your fingers, your back is too flat and most likely you have what is called a *posterior pelvis*. This type of posture causes your upper back to round forward excessively.

There are many more tests for posture,[35] so do a few and evaluate yourself.

Action Steps

Don't slouch when you're sitting. Sit straight and put your feet flat on the floor.

Get up and stretch often when you're working at your computer. Create a way to stand as an option to sitting when working. Alternate often and consciously.

Stand and walk straight: chin level to the ground, hips level.

Bring your phone up to your eye level; don't bend your neck down to look at it.

If you're struggling with back or neck pain because of poor posture, consider chiropractic adjustment or massage or yoga. All of these can help.

A Lower Level of Education

Several studies have shown that having less education is related to the risk of developing dementia.[36] In fact, the risk is nearly double for those with lower levels of education.

It appears that if you have a higher level of education, even if you do develop the plaques and tangles that are indicative of Alzheimer's, you are more able to retain cognitive function longer. You have more *cognitive reserve*, which simply means that your brain has adapted over time to create many connections between the cells. Instead of only one or two connections, you have 100 or 1,000 connections thanks to the learning you've done over the course of your life. If one or two connections are disrupted due to illness, toxic exposure, or Alzheimer's plaques, the other connections pick up the slack, so there is no disruption to the signal. But if you have only one or two connections, the signals can't get through and the symptoms of dementia show up.

This can be a difficult thing to overcome because many people do not have the opportunity for a higher education. My mom was yanked out of school in eighth grade to look after her older sister's children. Even though Mom was highly intelligent, she was unable, when confronted with her memory loss, to overcome it. Was that due to lack of cognitive reserve? Perhaps partially.

The good news is that you can do many things to make up for a lack of education. If you actively continue to learn things later in life, like a new language or to play a musical instrument, you can protect your brain against this risk factor. We'll discuss ways to do this in much more detail in chapter 16.

Early Retirement

Studies in the U.K.,[37] China,[38] and the European Union have all demonstrated that retirement accelerates the decline in verbal memory function, and delayed recall, which can be a predictor of dementia. The old saying "Use it or lose it" applies here. We'll be getting into many ways to keep your mind active and fresh in the second half of the book, but suffice it to say that you must keep your mind active if you want your brain to stay healthy.

Challenges Summary

As you've learned in these chapters, there are many factors that could increase your chances of developing any dementia, including Alzheimer's. Stress, lack of sleep, a poor diet, diabetes, depression, an unhealthy gut, lack of exercise, lack of social interaction – heck, even vision and hearing problems. Whew! The list seems overwhelming, doesn't it? I understand if you're feeling a bit overwhelmed with all this information. Where to start?

In the next chapter!

In this next segment of the book, we're going to get started on a logical, delicious program to save your brain and keep your precious memories intact.

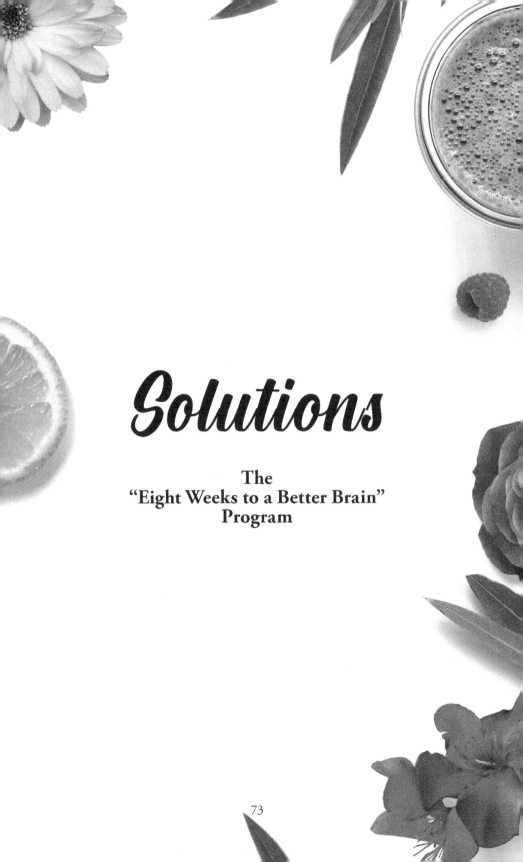

Solutions

The
"Eight Weeks to a Better Brain"
Program

Chapter 11

Introduction to the Program

From here on we'll be going step by step through the program to set you on a lifestyle course to eliminate or reduce your risk of developing dementia. These are incremental action steps that will take you from wherever you are now to a place where your health is optimized, your memories are sharp and clear, and your healthy brain can support you through all the wonderful things coming up in the rest of your life.

The program assumes a couple of things. First, that you're basically healthy, meaning you can shop, cook, do exercises, etc. Perhaps you have some "senior moments" now and again; you might even sometimes put your glasses in the fridge, but you can follow this program on your own.

I've designed the program to go from start to finish in about eight weeks, but you may take much longer, or you can speed through it. If you need to take two or three weeks to accomplish the goals for one week of the program, no problem. Or, if you're already doing many of the actions suggested in one segment and can merge two weeks together, that's okay, too.

Whatever it takes for you to accomplish this transformation is perfect, and however many actions you take is better than none. Dementia doesn't develop overnight, and you're not going to become the healthiest version of yourself overnight either.

All I ask is that you start sooner rather than later, because the changes that can lead to dementia may already be happening in your brain.

If you are starting the book here in order to begin the program right away, that means you haven't read about all the risk factors and why you're taking all these steps. That's no problem and I encourage you to start ASAP, but do go back to the whys in the first ten chapters as you're working through the program.

Understanding the reasons for doing everything you're doing will help you be even more motivated to stick with the program and follow through, and I want you to be as successful as possible.

We Are More Than Just Physical Beings

It's important to remember that we are much more than these physical bodies operated by a brain, muddling through the 80 or so years we have on Planet Earth. We are spiritual beings having a human experience, and all aspects of our being – body, mind, and spirit – are intimately connected. I call them the three pillars of health.

That's why, for every one of the eight weeks of this program, there are exercises, challenges, or action steps to support each of the pillars.

Do you have to do every one of them every week? Ideally that would be great, but we're all busy, and if you can only change or add one thing a week, that's okay. Just build on your successes and shrug off the things that didn't work. You can come back around and do them again later if you want to.

Remember, you don't have to do everything in this plan. And anything you do is better than nothing.

The Three Pillars

Body is about all the physical things that affect your brain. This is diet, detoxification, exercise, sleep, your environment, and even your hearing and oral health.

Mind is continual learning, stress management, enjoying time with others, and decluttering. Decluttering might seem like a physical thing, but it has as much, perhaps more, impact on your mind as it does on your body.

Spirit is listening to music, making music and dancing, learning an instrument, sound therapy, and, of course, the sounds of silence. Altruism, kindness, mindfulness, and some form of contemplative practice are also important aspects of this part of the plan.

The following is a summary of what you will be doing in the program. Details are addressed in the following chapters, and you will be prompted to refer back to previous chapters for information in case you've skipped directly to the program.

Body

1. Exercise

We're not talking marathons or endurance challenges here. We're talking 30 minutes of aerobic exercise at least five times a week. *Aerobic* means you get your heart pumping, which means you're oxygenating your brain (and everything else in your body); and you're working up a sweat, which helps your body detoxify.

If you can't fit in 30 minutes of walking all at once, break it up into three 10-minute walks. The goal is to make them brisk, but if you're just beginning to exercise, take your time to work up to that. Aim for 150 minutes per week by the end of these eight weeks.

If you don't exercise at all right now, this could be a bit of a challenge. But it is essential to try, so just start with a five-minute walk. Do a couple of trips up and down the stairs fast enough to make your breathing a little faster. Swim two or three laps. Whatever it is, get moving!

It's also important to be consistent, which means you need to be doing things you enjoy. There are many more exercise tips and suggestions in chapter 6, so go back to the "Action Steps" there if you're looking for other ideas.

2. Eat Well to Be Well

This, dear friend, means no processed foods. That means everything that comes in a box or package. This also means no bacon, pepperoni, ham, or "fake meat" burgers, and it means no fast food.

In this program, you cook. You are eating a whole-foods, plant-based diet. Everything I've learned over the last 10 years has led me to the conclusion that to keep our brains healthy, we should eliminate all animal products from our diets.

You will also drink lots of pure water. I don't mean bottled, because then you're getting the toxins from the plastic, and who knows whether or not the water in that bottle is as pure as they say it is? Purchase a good-quality water filter for your home system and take your water with you. Just be sure you drink plenty of it.

It's easy to remember: boxes, packages, and fast food – bad. Fresh, whole fruits; vegetables; seeds; and legumes – good.

In chapters 12 and 13 I include lists of foods to eat and foods to avoid, and in the appendix you'll find shopping lists, meal plans, and several recipes for brain-boosting meals. With these, you don't have to guess about what foods to eat, so it will be easier to stick with the plan.

3. Get Fresh Air and Sunshine

Fresh air and sunshine are essential for your health, especially for that of your brain. We did not evolve to work in artificial light. You need the rays of the sun and you need air that has not been recirculated.

4. Check your Hearing, Eyes, Teeth, Breathing, and Posture

You might or might not be able to get all of this done due to budgetary or logistical restraints, but if you feel that any of these are a problem, get them checked and treated. Read more about how to analyze and correct posture, ear, and eye issues in chapter 10.

If you have any reason to believe you're having breathing problems at night, get tested for sleep apnea. If you're not breathing properly, you might not get the right amount and type of sleep *and* you could be depriving your brain of oxygen.

5. Detoxify

It is as important to your health to detoxify your body as it is to eat and sleep well. If your body is filled with toxins, all your other efforts will not be as effective. (See chapter 7.) If you think you may be suffering from the effects of toxins, get tested so you'll know what you're dealing with, then you can do an effective detoxification program.

Over the course of this program you'll be taking steps to detoxify your home as best you can. That means getting rid of harsh chemical cleansers and getting a good air filter, at least for your bedroom.

6. Sleep

As mentioned in chapter 5, sleep issues contribute greatly to the likelihood of developing dementia, so it's important to get quality sleep. While common wisdom says we need eight hours per night, and that's a good number, what is even more important is that you go through all the *cycles* of sleep. Figure out how much sleep is optimal for you and stick to a sleep schedule. That means go to sleep and wake up at the same time every day (preferably with at least eight hours in that timeframe), even on weekends and holidays.

Mind

The pillar of *mind* involves continual learning, stress management, clearing your space, making, or listening to music, and spending quality time with others.

7. Declutter

Take inventory of your physical space. That includes home, workspace, even your automobile. Do you have a stationary bike sitting in a corner, covered in clothes? Is your kitchen counter so loaded up with papers and wrappings and dishes and kitsch that you must clean it off before even attempting to cook? When you begin a new journey, it's helpful to have a clean slate.

Check your pantry. What in there is processed, canned, or boxed? If you are in a financial position to do so, donate those items to a food bank. (I know… it's like passing off bad food; but something is better than nothing.)

If you just can't part with these foods, put them in order of what needs to be eaten first and intersperse them with the good fresh foods you're going to be preparing during this journey. Hopefully this won't last more than a week because we need to get your body cleaned out for this process to work. That said, I am not keen on waste, so do whatever you feel is right for you to get your food pantry in order.

The same goes for your bathroom and under the sink in your kitchen. A jug of vinegar, baking soda, and some essential oils are all you need for cleaning. (See the recipes in the appendix.) Get rid of everything else in an environmentally safe manner.

Clean everything that you haven't worn for a year from your closet (unless it's a size smaller than you currently are, because you're probably going to lose some weight on this program). When I did this, I passed on to thrift stores more than half of my wardrobe. It is very freeing, and it helps set up your mind for the "new you."

Clear off your desk, your dresser, the chair in your bedroom. Make your bedroom a Zen space for good sleep. Clutter there can make it difficult to turn off your mind and get a good night's sleep.

These can be done little by little as you're changing your eating and exercise habits. Decluttering is very inspirational: clear space, clear mind.

8. Learn Something New

There are many suggestions for this in chapter 16, including learning a new language or a musical instrument. Travel to a new place, even if it's just a state or province away. Read a book about a topic that interests you but is different from anything you would have read or studied in the past.

If there's something you've always wanted to learn or do – do it! Many people take up painting or quilting or knitting later in life. Go for it! And if you do it with other people, all the better. Which leads us to the next step.

9. Spend Quality Social Time with Others

I say "quality time" because spending time with others who are not supportive of you is not good for your mind or your brain. However, a rich social life is a powerful defense against dementia. (See chapter 9.)

If you like to sing, join a choir. If you already play a musical instrument, form a band or ensemble with friends. Or take dance lessons. Not only is it a great social activity, it is one of the best exercises you can do.

Join a book club; or if you go to church, get involved with a group there. Besides protecting your brain, you might just make some amazing friends and learn some great new things.

10. Listen To and/or Make Music, Sing, and Dance

The benefits of making music cannot be overstated, so if it is at all possible, take up some kind of instrument or sing. Just remember that it is the act of learning and playing that you're aiming for here. It's not about being a master. The goal is to enjoy the process of creating music. It does not mean performing. We'll discuss all of this in chapter 18.

Listen to music whenever and wherever you can. Whether it's attending a live classical concert, listening to recordings of Johnny Mathis, walking to jazzy music, or experiencing vibroacoustic therapy, music is not only a powerful preventive, it also helps slow down the progress of cognitive decline and can even reverse it once it has begun. You'll learn more about this in chapter 17.

Dancing is a great exercise, so there's that – but it is also a great social activity, and the complex movements required for dances like salsa are excellent for your mind.

Spirit

Spirit is all those things that inspire and nurture us. Music fulfills this need as well, but here you will add other things that inspire you to kindness, generosity, and love toward others. This is important because your brain responds to altruism and love. You are wired to be a spiritual being, and attending to that is vital for your health.

11. Meditation and Mindfulness

Meditation is one of the greatest protectors we have against stress, but it is also directly correlated to a healthier brain and a greater sense of peace and self.

Over the past decade, scientific evidence has been accumulating that shows that meditation can help us maintain healthier brains and bodies as we age.

This is an integral part of this program, and even if you have never meditated before, you can take advantage of its amazing power simply by mindfully breathing. Take five minutes to sit quietly and pay attention to your breath.

Mindfulness means doing tasks with focused intent. It is the opposite of attempting to do the impossible… multitasking. In this eight-week program you take one attribute of mindfulness each week and incorporate it into your daily life.

Yoga, qigong, and tai chi, while excellent exercise for your body, are also powerful tools for centering your mind and getting in touch with your soul. For many people who have trouble sitting still, these kinds of moving meditation are great ways to get used to the whole idea of meditation.

12. **Painting, Writing, and Other Creative Pursuits**

Whether or not you have ever thought of yourself as creative, one of the most powerful things you can do to save your brain is to express yourself. Whether that is with paint or by sketching, writing, knitting, or creating beautiful quilts, the act of creating something opens up a channel from your inner self to the outer world. Fears, hopes, desires, and many other emotions can be expressed, helping heal and nurture your spiritual self. Connecting with your inner self opens you up to more meaningful relationships with others.

Expressing yourself in creative ways stimulates neuroplasticity by creating new channels of communication between neurons. I discuss this at great length in chapter 18, so be sure to consider this an important part of saving your brain and not something to be relegated to "some time, when I have time."

13. **Generosity, Kindness, and Your Spiritual Self**

We are not just the sum of our parts, bundles of neurons and cells organized in organs and systems directed by the master controller, our brain. We are spiritual beings having this human experience, and we are social animals, dependent on our interactions with others.

The feel-good effects of generosity are triggered by changes in brain chemistry that occur when you give. Several different "happiness chemicals" are produced, including dopamine and endorphins, which give people a sense of euphoria. Oxytocin, which is associated with tranquility, serenity, or inner peace, is also produced.

The connection to brain health has been revealed in several studies that show that giving time and assistance to others reduces stress, which we know is a huge risk factor for dementia.

Kindness and gratitude are powerful traits that help us keep our brains whole and our minds sharp. By nurturing others and our own spirituality, we are much healthier, because while our genes are the blueprints for our lives, we are the architects. Read more about this in chapter 20.

Dr. Bruce Lipton reminds us in his work on epigenetics that we are not at the mercy of our physiology. Our minds, both conscious and subconscious, determine how our genes express themselves. By knowing this, and by connecting to our spiritual selves, we have incredible power over our health, including the health of our brains.

In this program you are encouraged to take the time to nurture a contemplative practice and consider your place in the world, your mission, and your purpose.

The Weekly Plan

As we go forward, remember that imperfect completion is better than never starting. You do not have to do everything in this program to get some benefit, and certainly not all at once. Have fun as you embark on this wonderful journey that will protect your memories and help you be healthier and more energetic.

When I created this program, I was a vegetarian who loved potato chips. If you come to the program as a dyed-in-the-wool carnivore who loves milkshakes, this transformation might be a bit harder for you than it was for me, and you will likely have to go a little more slowly because you will be spending more time initially on eliminating those things.

It doesn't matter. Start wherever you come into the picture. If you're already exercising but are still eating cheese – start by eliminating cheese. If you're addicted to the standard American diet (SAD), and you haven't had more exercise than it takes to get from your couch to your car, then start by walking around the block.

This is a lifestyle change, and it is not going to happen overnight. And you will likely slide backward from time to time. I certainly did. That's okay. Just be kind and patient, but be persistent.

The following chart shows the steps to be taken in each of the next eight weeks (or longer if you need more time!) Remember, this is the "ideal" that incorporates all the components of this program. You might or might not get to all of them each week, but I encourage you to celebrate your milestones. We all deserve a pat on the back from time to time, especially from ourselves!

In the appendix you will find the recipes and references you'll need to follow the plan, plus many extras. Remember also to refer to the chapters that are noted on the chart to clarify any actions that you're not certain about.

It might look like a lot, and it is, but every step is easy. There is nothing complicated (except maybe some of the cooking if you're not used to it).

Be sure to keep a journal so you'll be able to set some goals and reflect on your journey. It's also a great way to keep track of recipes that you like (or don't!)

Week One

Body: First Steps: Bye, Bye, Sugar – Chapter 4

This first week is about working to eliminate sugar and anything with artificial sweeteners. Read labels! Check everything in your cupboards and fridge and eliminate everything that has sugar, aspartame, or sucralose in the ingredient list. You can also start eliminating processed foods because they likely include sugar.

You're going to satisfy your sweet tooth with yummy smoothies and there are even some tasty desserts in this week's meal plan.

Exercise – Chapter 6

This week and every week, exercise is a must. If you've been mostly sedentary, this week is all about getting started. Walk as much as you can, preferably outside. If you normally exercise, keep it up. The goal is 30 minutes a day, six days a week.

Mind: Make the Commitment; Set Daily Goals

This week you're starting a new lifestyle. It's not easy to see where all this is going, so having daily goals is helpful, as is keeping a journal. Try something like "Just for today, I will not eat any donuts."

Take a few moments and write out why it is important for you to be doing this program. This will help you stay focused on the end result, which makes it easier to make the healthier choices.

Spirit: Begin Meditation – Chapter 20

Meditation is a powerful stress-reducing, intention-focusing tool that you will be using throughout this program. If you are a beginner you might enjoy the guided meditation in the appendix, or simply sit quietly, paying attention to your breathing, for five minutes.

If you have trouble with sitting meditation, consider a walking meditation (more about that in chapter 20) or qigong. There is a reference to a free qigong class in the appendix.

Advanced: If you've already been meditating, continue your normal practice.

Mindfulness Focus this Week – *Beginner's Mind:* Try to look at everything as if for the very first time – the joy, the feeling, the uniqueness of every moment and every experience.

Week Two
Ongoing: Eliminating sugar and processed foods. Continue meditation and exercise.
Body: Chapter 3   This week you're also going to say "so long" to animal products, or at least start this process. This will likely take a while, perhaps even the duration of this program if you're a cheese lover, but your gut (and your waistline) will thank you.   **Planning Ahead** – Make sauerkraut to use in Week 4. The recipe is in the appendix. If this is not something you have time for or are prepared to do, you can source sauerkraut or kimchi in the deli section of your grocery so you will have it for Week 4.   **Exercise** – Every day, try to walk a little farther and/or a little faster. The goal, by the end of the eight-week program, is to walk briskly for 30 minutes at 100 paces per minute. This is achieved more easily if you have music to help you along (chapter 6).
Mind: Declutter, Chapter 10, and Detoxify, Chapter 7   To keep your mind clear and focused, it helps to clear out your space, which includes the kitchen and bathroom. This will be ongoing, but for this week, start by getting rid of the toxic chemicals that are lurking under your kitchen sink and in your bathrooms. Replace the cleaners with ones you can make using the recipes in the appendix or online, or *carefully* shop for natural, non-toxic cleaners and personal-care products.
Spirit: After meditation, consider making notes about how you're feeling. Are you noticing anything different about how you react to stress or are you feeling more clarity?   If you feel ready, consider yoga. In the appendix is a reference to a great, simple yoga video with stretches and breathing. Just 10 minutes can make a huge difference to start your day.   **Mindfulness Focus this Week** – *Non-Judging*: Try to see what it feels like to just be an impartial witness instead of judging people and events that come up every day.

Week Three
Ongoing: Continue to eliminate sugar and processed foods, to meditate, and to exercise. Continue eliminating toxins from the kitchen and bathroom. If you've started yoga or tai chi or qigong, continue. Consistency is important.
Body: Improve Gut Health – Chapter 3 This week's meal plan adds kombucha tea, your first fermented food. You can buy kombucha in most grocery stores and certainly in health food stores. Start slowly, just 4 ounces a day. If you have not already done it, this week aim to eliminate dairy products. This is hard for many people, so try integrating your recipes with Vegan Cheese and/or Vegan Butter and Vegan "Alfredo" Sauce to ease the transition. The detoxification goal this week is to evaluate your cookware – no PTFE or aluminum (chapter 7). **Exercise** – If you're building up the walking pace and duration, keep at it. Make yourself breathless from time to time. Start working on building leg strength.
Mind: Stress Reduction – Chapter 8 This week evaluate sources of stress and review the many stress-reduction techniques in chapter 8. Institute as many as you can, including mindful music listening and getting outside. Qigong, tai chi, and yoga are also all good for stress. Try one of these at least a couple of days this week.
Spirit: A Spiritual Practice Makes a Huge Difference – Chapters 18 and 20 Take time this week to think about who it is you want to be. Where do you want to be in five years? Are you excited about anything? If not, why not? What can you do to inspire yourself – maybe writing or art? Have you been neglecting a spiritual practice? Perhaps consider revisiting it. Or volunteer. **Mindfulness Focus this Week** – *Patience:* Try to let everything unfold in its time; don't be in a hurry to get through one thing in order to move on to the next one.

Week Four
Ongoing: Exercise and meditation continue for the duration. Sugar and processed food should be eliminated now, and you're eliminating toxins from kitchen and bathroom. Reducing inflammation is a continued theme this week (chapter 3).
Body: Focus on gut health with kombucha, and add at least one forkful a day of sauerkraut or kimchi. Work up to 8 ounces of kombucha per day.   Add prebiotics in the form of veggies (chapter 12) to feed the probiotics in the fermented foods. Dairy products and eggs should be eliminated by the end of this week.   Continue detoxification by checking your diet for other sources of toxins like heavy metals, phthalates from plastic, and others outlined in chapter 7. Scan for hearing and tooth problems (chapter 10).   **Exercise** – If it is not already added, try to do strength training a couple of days a week.
Mind: Learn Something New – Chapter 16   For the rest of your life you should be learning something new every day. That could be auditing a university course or taking one of the thousands of online offerings.   Consider learning a musical instrument, or study a new language. These are the most powerful brain-enhancing activities. Decide this week what it is you're going to learn first, enroll, and get started.   Spend time in silence and purposefully listen to music (chapter 17).
Spirit: Hopefully you can sit in meditation or something similar for 15 minutes or more now. If you are struggling, you may enjoy guided meditations. Or simply try mindfully breathing for just two or three minutes per day.   Another great way to connect with your spirit and the spirit of the planet is to get outside in the sunshine and walk barefoot (depending on safety and season, of course). In addition to the physical, bioelectrical benefits of grounding, or *earthing*, it is also powerful for stress reduction and overall health.   **Mindfulness Focus this Week** – *Trust:* Strive to pay attention to self-doubting thoughts when they arise and look deeply into where they really come from instead of believing them. Trust yourself.

Week Five
Ongoing: Ensure that dairy products, sugar, and processed foods are eliminated and continue to monitor for toxins in your house and food. Continue with sauerkraut and kombucha.
Body: Time-Restricted Eating – Chapter 14 If you have a few extra pounds to shed, this week you're going to work on that because you'll be going into a mild state of ketosis. At the same time, you'll be cleaning out old and damaged brain cells with fasting and ketosis. First step: a 12-hour fast. If you finish your last meal at 6:30 p.m., don't eat anything else until at least 6:30 the next morning. Do that at least five days this week. Try incorporating coconut oil in your diet from now on, as it helps you get into a state of ketosis, which does wonders for the brain.
Mind: Chapter 11 This week, as you're cleaning out your brain through fasting, you will also clean out more of the clutter in your home, office, and mind. Hopefully as you've eliminated sugar and processed foods from your diet, you've removed those packages from your cupboards. If not, now is the time to do it. Same process for the fridge. Clean out your closet, your dresser, the chair in your bedroom. Make your bedroom a Zen space for good sleep.
Spirit: New this week: Mindfully listening to silence and to music, focusing on how it feeds your soul (chapter 17). Go online and listen to some of the music of your youth. Make a note in your journal – how did this make you feel? Did it inspire you to connect with someone? Did it trigger any other memories? **Mindfulness Focus this Week** – *Non-Striving:* Don't feel you have to always "do it right". If you do, you will always be questioning yourself and not actually enjoying what you are doing or experiencing.

Week Six
Ongoing: Continuing with meditation and exercise, and no dairy products, sugar, or processed foods. Continue eating sauerkraut or kimchi and drinking kombucha every day. Five days at least of time-restricted eating continues for this week.
Body: Sleep – Chapter 5 Are you getting seven to eight hours of sleep per night? By now your gut should be in fairly good shape, and sleeping should be better. If you do have trouble getting a good night's sleep, be sure to go over the steps in chapter 5. If necessary, consider a supplement like melatonin or valerian root. One great way to help get a good night's sleep is with aromatherapy. See chapter 15 for some ideas about the best scents to use for relaxation and sleep. You've been enjoying this new lifestyle for six weeks now, so you should be experiencing some changes in your digestion, less inflammation in your joints, less swelling in your feet and hands, and hopefully less stress. Do an assessment.
Mind: Sing, Dance, Listen to Music – Chapter 18 It's time to play some music this week. Pick up that old guitar in the corner. Or dust off the piano and play. Or buy a djembe and join a drumming circle. Beat on a bowl with a couple of wooden spoons. Go dancing. Sing. If you're able to sing in a choir, all the better. It is a wonderful way to get the benefits of the mathematics of music and the social interaction that is so important to your brain health.
Spirit: Kindness and Generosity and the Spiritual Self – Chapter 20 Is there somewhere you can volunteer or help others this week? Making a difference in the world, whether it's for animal welfare (being vegan is a big part of that!), helping refugees, or volunteering to teach English or math, is good for your brain. **Mindfulness Focus this Week –** *Acceptance:* Accept where you are, how you are. No one ever changed by hating themselves into it.

Week Seven
Ongoing: Continue with exercise, meditation, fermented foods, and time-restricted eating with at least 12 hours off.
Body: Inflammation and the Immune System – Chapter 3 Aim for seven days of time-restricted eating this week. If you're doing well with the 12 hours on and 12 hours off, you can add one or two days of 14 hours off and 10 hours of eating per day. Review how well you've done eliminating inflammatory foods. Ideally now you should also be steering away from alcohol (you should find you don't crave it with the other changes going on), and talk to your doctor if you're on any prescription medications. Could they be causing any inflammation? Add more spices and foods that protect against it and ensure that you are eating the fermented foods and prebiotics. **Exercise –** Aim for 150 minutes of aerobic exercise per week plus two days of strength and/or resistance training.
Mind: Improve Social Connections – Chapter 9 Take time this week to consciously connect with those who have been important in your life. Share memories with them, have a laugh, or a good cry. Do something new or different with those you see often. Explore a new place or try new foods. These new things create new pathways in your brain.
Spirit: Creativity, Your Spirit, and Your Brain – Chapter 18 In our busy lives it's quite easy to ignore those creative inklings we've had for years. Busy careers, raising children, keeping house – all these things take us away from the part of us that would like to express feelings, ideas, hopes, and dreams. *Now* is the time to explore these feelings, because drawing, writing, painting, needlework… any creative pursuit is not only good for your brain, it's good for your soul. Happy soul, happy brain. **Mindfulness Focus this Week –** *Letting go*: of judgment, striving, and expectations in order to make room for joy and acceptance.

Week Eight
Ongoing: Continue detoxing your home and your body. Continue exercise and meditation, fermented foods, and time-restricted eating. Keep learning.
Body: Set the Stage for the Rest of Your Life There are many complementary and experimental therapies discussed in chapter 19. As you continue your new healthy lifestyle, you may want to explore some of them. If you're still having some memory issues or trouble with sleep, light therapy and vibro-acoustic therapy can be immensely helpful. Go back to your notes or journal and take an inventory of how you have been feeling as these eight weeks have progressed. Is inflammation down? Do you have more energy? Finally – holidays are a difficult time when you're just starting a plant-based diet, so see the appendix for some simple vegan recipes for special occasions.
Mind: Keep It Simple Your space is hopefully now decluttered and your mind can focus without distractions. Now aim to *keep* your cupboards and your mind that way. Happiness is not a loaded shopping cart. Minimalism is an honorable goal. With every choice, whether it's buying something or eating something, ask yourself this question: "Is this good for my brain?" Evaluate all the things you enjoy that can enhance neuroplasticity and continued growth. Keep doing them and always explore new ways to engage your mind.
Spirit: As you go forward with your new lifestyle, continue to explore and nurture what matters to you. What fulfills your spiritual self? What do you value most in your life? What inspires you and gives you hope? What brings you joy? What are your proudest achievements? What would you like to achieve in the future? As you become more self-aware, check in with yourself often because it will help you stay on track for your physical, emotional, and spiritual health.

Chapter 12

Foods to Eat, and Why

Thankfully, it is incredibly simple to eat a brain-healthy diet: Fresh. Whole. Organic whenever possible. Plant-based.

All the foods listed here are included because there is research supporting their value for brain health, and I didn't list anything that I don't personally eat or that I don't recommend to my clients.

Throughout this chapter are references to the many recipes in the appendix. They are provided so you don't have to come up with ways to use these foods at first. Start with the recipes I included, then go online from there. The possibilities are endless!

Vegetables

Basically all vegetables are good for your brain. They have fiber, which is essential to gut health, and they are full of antioxidants and phytonutrients, which help protect your brain. But it is important that you eat organic. Conventionally grown vegetables also serve up big portions of herbicides and pesticides. Two of the healthiest leafy green vegetables, spinach and kale, were numbers two and three on the Environmental Working Group's list of "Dirty Dozen"[1] fruits and vegetables for 2019.

Due to budgetary and availability constraints, many of us cannot buy organic all the time, but do try to buy organic. The Environmental Working Group also has a "Clean Fifteen" list, so if you are watching your budget, you know that those non-organic products are a bit safer to eat.

The one exception to eating as many vegetables as you can is white potatoes. While they contain generous amounts of vitamin B_6, potassium, copper, vitamin C, manganese, phosphorus, niacin, dietary fiber, and pantothenic acid, they are also high in starch. Starch, of course, turns quickly into sugars in your body.

Cruciferous

Broccoli, cauliflower, cabbage, and Brussels sprouts all contain sulforaphane, which helps reduce inflammation. Since inflammation is a huge contributor to dementia, these are great additions to your diet. *Plus* you are adding fiber to help your gut.

Cabbage is especially beneficial for its anti-inflammatory effects. The anthocyanin in cabbage, particularly red cabbage (also called purple cabbage), helps reduce inflammation. Red cabbage is high in the B vitamins, which help nourish and support the nervous system, help restore nerve cells, and improve blood supply to the brain. Red cabbage also contains vitamin K, which aids in the production of the myelin sheath,[2] which protects nerves from damage and decay.

Cabbage and Brussels sprouts also contain the omega-3 fatty acid alpha-linolenic acid (ALA).

Leafy Greens

Kale and spinach have large amounts of B_6 and B_{12} vitamins, and kale is also high in vitamin K, which, besides protecting the myelin sheath, is essential for verbal memory.[3]

Beets

The fiber found in beets aids in the reduction of cholesterol and triglycerides by increasing high-density lipoproteins (HDL) – the "good" cholesterol. Beets also contain a nutrient called betaine, which lowers your level of homocysteine, which is bad for blood vessels. Beets have been found to help prevent atherosclerosis, heart attacks, and strokes, all drivers of the path to dementia. One study even found that consuming beet juice for just one week helped dramatically reduce blood pressure!

Beets are high in potassium, and the carbohydrates found in beets are natural building blocks of energy metabolism while causing no negative side effects like other high-carbohydrate foods. The vitamin A and lutein in beets also help keep your eyes healthy.

Eat as much as you like, but a couple of times a week would be great. There is a recipe for pickled beets in the appendix because it is one of the favorite ways to consume beets. They are also fantastic in morning smoothies. And the greens are edible too!

> *A word of caution about beets: Beet greens contain high levels of oxalate, which might contribute to the creation of kidney stones. And consuming large amounts of beets has been linked to gout. If you're predisposed to those issues, you should probably steer away. Don't worry if your urine or stool is red or pink after eating beets — that's just the expelling process of the color.*

Garlic

Garlic's antiseptic properties help support its reputation for fighting colds. Garlic plays a role in lowering cholesterol and triglycerides, increasing circulation, and protecting blood vessels from inflammation.[4] It has also been shown to prevent the death of neurons, and helps improve learning and memory retention.[5]

The health benefits of garlic are enhanced further when a garlic clove is chopped, crushed, or chewed, releasing the powerful sulfur compounds within. If you wait 10 minutes after chopping or crushing, you will release more of the compounds that are so valuable. Garlic is also a great source of prebiotics.

Eat as much as you can in anything you can. Most of the recipes in this book use garlic.

Onions

Onions aid digestion through a special carbohydrate called fructo-oligosaccharides (FOS).[6] It is essentially a prebiotic that feeds the good bacteria in your gut and fights off the bad bacteria. It also helps improve digestive function by aiding bowel movements.

Onions are also great for the immune system and are powerful when you are detoxifying. And there have been studies that showed their value in helping the brain recover after stroke or clots[7] – both of which can contribute to dementia.

So, like garlic, eat onions as much as you can. In our home we literally eat them both every day.

Sea Vegetables and Seaweed

If you are a fan of sushi, then you are familiar with at least one kind of sea-weed – nori. But there are about 10,000 species including spirulina and kelp. Sea vegetables are chock full of nutrients. They have minerals including calcium, copper, and iron. They are rich in vitamins, specifically vitamin K and folic acid, and are good sources of protein and fiber.

Seaweed is high in glutamate, an amino acid necessary for normal brain function.[8]

Sea vegetables are also a good source of iodine, selenium, and tyrosine, which are important for healthy thyroid function. When your thyroid is underactive, memory problems, inattention, and depression can occur.[9] An overactive thyroid can lead to anxiety and sleeplessness.

Research shows that a brown seaweed called fucoxanthin can help improve insulin resistance and blood-sugar control.[10]

> *A word of warning: If you are taking blood-thinning medications, be cautious with sea vegetables because of the high vitamin K content. If you're taking thyroid medications, you should talk to your doctor before adding a lot of seaweed to your diet.*

Another problem with seaweed is the fact that it comes from one of the most polluted places on the planet – the ocean. Heavy metals and chemicals like mercury, cadmium, lead, and arsenic can be present in large numbers in anything from the sea. A little seaweed can be beneficial, so don't refuse it because of the dangers of the ocean; just be aware that like sea salt, it can contain unhealthy components that are, unfortunately, part of our oceans.

Sprouts

These are seeds that have been allowed to germinate into young plants. They are more nutritious than the nut, seed, vegetable, grain, or legume that has sprouted. They also contain lower levels of antinutrients, which means it's easier for your body to absorb the nutrients. Studies have shown that sprouts can help people with type 2 diabetes control their blood sugar.

You might have heard of some cases of food poisoning from sprouts that have not been germinated or stored properly, and that is one of the reasons I grow my own. It's amazingly easy, and much less expensive than buying them in the grocery store. (You're also not contributing to the plastic pollution problem when you make your own.) I use just a couple of drops of food-grade hydrogen peroxide in the initial soaking, and control the temperature and humidity to ensure that there is no chance of salmonella or E. coli taking up residence. You can get sprouting seeds and supplies online, and it's easy to find organic sources.

Sweet Potatoes

These amazing tubers come in yellow, orange, and purple, so they have varying amounts of vitamin A, which helps your cells communicate and grow better, and B_6, which is an essential coenzyme for cognitive development. Potassium and magnesium are also plentiful, which supports healthy blood pressure and leads to a healthier heart. All sweet potatoes are also high in fiber, which is essential for bodily functions, especially maintaining a healthy weight and fighting type 2 diabetes.

There are literally thousands of amazing recipes using sweet potatoes, but one of the tastiest also incorporates the inflammation-reducing spices ginger, turmeric, and pepper. I've included the recipe for my favorite Sweet Potato Anti-Inflammatory Muffins in the appendix.

Mushrooms

Mushrooms are not vegetables (they're fungi), but they are super nutritious and are eaten in mostly the same ways as vegetables. Studies have shown that eating more than two portions of cooked mushrooms per week could lead to a 50 percent lower risk of mild cognitive impairment (MCI),[11] which can lead to Alzheimer's.

A standard portion is ¾ of a cup, or about 150 grams. They can be dried or packaged, and any variety is beneficial. Almost all contain ergothioneine, which is an anti-inflammatory antioxidant believed to be the reason for mushrooms' powerful anti-dementia benefits.

Lion's mane mushrooms are particularly powerful. These are 20 percent protein and contain many potent brain-enhancing compounds. They've been shown to activate the peptide known as *nerve growth factor*, which is necessary for the growth, maintenance, and survival of neurons.

It's best to eat mushrooms cooked, and there are so many easy recipes that you won't have any trouble finding something you like. I include a few recipes in the appendix, but your imagination is the only limit to the delicious ways you can incorporate them into your diet.

Probiotics and Fermented Foods

There is a large body of evidence that shows the value of fermented foods for maintaining cognitive health. A powerful meta-study of 45 research projects confirmed that fermented foods ranging from ginseng root to cabbage to rice are all powerful brain enhancers and savers.[12]

When you are introducing these powerful foods to your body, you should do so slowly. One tablespoon of sauerkraut on a salad. Four ounces of kombucha tea. Even kefir water, which is very mild, takes getting used to. But don't let that scare you off. They are essential to gut health, and most people have no problems. Just take it slow and easy. In the program we start with just four ounces of kombucha a day for a week and go from there.

If you have stomach issues, be sure to consult with your naturopath or integrative practitioner to see which fermented foods to choose, and how much and how fast to add them to your regimen.

It's easy to make your own fermented foods. Beets, cabbage, tomatoes, onions, garlic, and green beans are just a few of the veggies you can use. It's very inexpensive and surprisingly easy. Recipes for sauerkraut and kimchi are included under "Vegan Basics" in the appendix. It's especially important to buy organic produce to make your fermented food. In addition to avoiding the pesticides, this produce should come from healthy soil because that will give you more of the microbes needed to create a more valuable fermented product.

You can certainly buy fermented products at most natural food stores and some supermarkets. Fermented foods are full of live organisms that must be kept cool to survive, so choose fermented items only from the refrigerated section of the store. Tempeh, tofu, natto, and miso are fermented, but be sure they are made with non-GMO soy.

Yogurt made from plant milk is filled with probiotics, so you can have that tasty treat without the dangers of dairy products. I make coconut milk yogurt, which is incredibly easy if you have a slow cooker or instant pot. There's also a recipe for that under "Vegan Basics."

Apple cider vinegar is one of the most widely used fermented products. Many of the recipes in this book utilize it, as the acetic acid helps stimulate production of the enzymes needed to break down fats.

Fruits

The more, the merrier, but there is research showing that the ones discussed below are especially good for brain health.

Apples

This common fruit contains many antioxidants[13] including quercetin, which has a neuroprotective effect.[14] In a 2015 mouse study, high doses of quercetin appeared to help protect cells from the type of damage that can lead to Alzheimer's disease.[15]

It has been found that the average apple contains about 100 million bacteria of various species. Most are inside, not on the skin. These bacteria join and interact with the trillions of microbes that are already in your gut and help your gut biome become even more diverse and valuable to your brain.

Most of the microbes happen to be in the core, which is also full of fiber. While apple seeds contain trace amounts of cyanide, adults are not likely to have any adverse effects from eating a core once a day. It might sound weird to eat the core of the apple, but your gut will thank you. One easy way to do that is to just throw the whole apple into your smoothie.

Avocados

Truly a superfood, avocados are powerhouses of nutrition. They improve blood supply and oxygenation to your brain, and their monounsaturated fatty acids help protect nerve cells, which provide support to information-carrying nerves. They also contain folate, which is essential for brain health and the maintenance of cognitive function, including memory.

What's in an avocado? One-half of an avocado provides nearly 3.5 grams of soluble and insoluble fiber to keep the digestive system happy. It also contains oleic acid, which is a fat that activates the part of your brain that makes you feel full; lots of potassium and vitamins E and C; and other nutrients that help reduce inflammation.

Eat at least ½ an avocado per day.

Berries

Berries contain flavonoids that can improve numerous cognitive skills including memory, learning, and decision-making. They can also prevent age-related mental decline and protect against Alzheimer's disease.[16] Blueberries are one of the best sources of these great flavonoids.

Berries are also full of antioxidants that neutralize the free radicals that can damage brain cells. It's wise to eat berries at least a couple of times a week. Frozen varieties are fine.

Bananas

Bananas are high in antioxidants and contain serotonin, which improves memory and learning. They also contain a high amount of dopamine, which can boost attention and memory, and are a great source of vitamin B_6, magnesium, and the amino acids tryptophan and tyrosine, which your body uses to make the neurotransmitters serotonin and dopamine.

Did you know you can also eat banana peels? They have more tryptophan than is found in the fruit and are also richer in both soluble and insoluble fiber than the banana itself. You can eat the peels as a fried or dried treat, or you can add them to the blender when making a smoothie or juice. Just be sure to buy organic, because conventionally grown bananas are sprayed many times during the growth cycle. You can also steam the peel and make it into a tea. You'll find many recipes online.

Cacao

Yes, cacao is a fruit. And what a fruit! Cacao flavanols facilitate brain-cell connections and survival, and protect brain cells from toxins and the negative effects of inflammation. Cacao is one of the richest sources of antioxidants on the planet and has been shown to increase blood flow to the brain. In one study people who consumed medium and high amounts of these flavanols every day made significant improvements on tests that measured attention, executive function, and memory.[17]

The best way to reap the benefits is from a powder that is as natural as possible and has not been chemically processed and roasted. Raw organic cacao is also one of the best plant-based sources of magnesium, which helps turn glucose into energy.

Studies suggest that a daily intake of 200 mg of cacao flavanols is a potential target. *Cocoa* is made from roasted beans (and usually added ingredients), while *cacao*, which is what I'm promoting here, has not been roasted or added to.

Dates

The soluble fiber in dates helps keep your digestive system operating correctly, and dates help create good bacteria in your stomach to nurture the all-important microbiome.

These tasty fruits are easily incorporated into smoothies and are excellent snacks. They are high in calories and natural sugars, though, so eat them sparingly. One or two a day is sufficient.

Olives

Olives contain monounsaturated fatty acids, which are linked with lowering LDL ("bad" cholesterol) while maintaining HDL ("good" cholesterol"). Because of their polyphenols, they also help reduce oxidative stress caused by inflammation and protect the tissues of vital organs like your brain from harmful and potentially irreversible damage. Olives also contain vitamin E, which is linked to improved cognition and reduced risk of cognitive decline.

Plantains

Plantains[18] provide many vitamins and minerals and can be a great substitute for rice or potatoes. They contain high levels of magnesium, which is important in regulating blood pressure; potassium; and vitamin B_6, which encourages the production of norepinephrine and serotonin, chemical messengers that help keep the mind stable. They also contain homocysteine, an amino acid that keeps the nervous system and blood vessels healthy. High in vitamin C and vitamin A, they are also powerful immune-system boosters.

Plantains control blood glucose by improving carbohydrate metabolism while regulating insulin. This reduces your chances of developing type 2 diabetes.

If you haven't tried plantains yet – do. You can just boil them and eat them like potatoes, but there are thousands of different ways to enjoy these fiber-rich fruits. You can use them as a stuffing in wraps, or even make them into "chips" (not the healthiest way to use them, but delicious). I included a couple of recipes in the "International Flavors" section because they are so healthy, and not something most North Americans would normally have in their diet.

Red Grapes

Red grapes contain resveratrol, which you've no doubt heard is the reason that red wine is supposed to be so healthy. (One small glass per day.)

Red grapes can enhance brain health and delay the onset of degenerative neural diseases. In one study published in the *British Journal of Nutrition*, it was shown that grape juice can improve the brain function of older people who have already displayed MCI.[19]

Drinking red grape juice is one way to get the benefits, but the best is to eat them, since you also get all the other nutrients and fiber in the whole fruit. Eat organic, though, because conventionally grown grapes are sprayed mercilessly with serious amounts of pesticides.

One study found that about 2¼ cups of grapes per day was the most beneficial for health.

Beverages

Coffee

Several studies have shown that drinking coffee every day could help fight off dementia. In one study researchers looked at the caffeine consumption of 6,500 women aged between 65 and 80 and found that those who consumed more than 261 mg of caffeine a day had a 36 percent lower chance of getting dementia.[20] That would be about three cups of coffee or six cups of black tea.

In another study researchers at Stanford found that caffeine can help lower inflammation,[21] which in one way or another is behind most cases of Alzheimer's and other chronic diseases. Older participants who drank more caffeinated beverages had less inflammation in their bodies. Subsequent laboratory tests showed that it was the caffeine that was protecting them. So a moderate amount of caffeinated coffee is, like tea, protective against dementia. Choose organic if possible.

Chemically decaffeinated coffee is problematic, because when you add chemicals to any process, you're adding hazards. Removing the caffeine also removes its neuroprotective benefits. If caffeine keeps you awake, try coffee that's been decaffeinated using a water process rather than a chemical process.

Tea

Frequent tea drinking is associated with a lower risk of dementia.[22] Findings suggest that the brain-protecting effects of tea likely stem from the bioactive compounds in the leaves. Those include flavonoids, which have anti-inflammatory and antioxidant potential, and L-theanine, which regulates neurotransmitter and brain activities.

A double-blind placebo-controlled study showed that a combination of green tea extract and L-theanine improved memory and attention in subjects with MCI.[23] Another study involving subjects with no cognition problems showed that just a single dose of matcha tea induced slight improvements in speed of attention and episodic secondary memory.[24]

In one study, people who ate more foods with the antioxidant flavanol, which is found in tea, were 48 percent less likely to later develop Alzheimer's than those who consumed fewer flavanols from all sources, after adjusting for other factors that could affect the risk of Alzheimer's.[25]

Green tea – especially the extract, or matcha – seems to be the best for protecting the brain and for improving memory and cognition, but black tea is also beneficial. Many herbal teas are polyphenol powerhouses.

A warning is warranted here: In the last couple of years researchers have found pesticide residues in many teas, even high-end brands. Check online to see where your brand stands.[26]

Water

You must be adequately hydrated for your brain to operate at its optimal level. But as I mentioned in chapter 7, much of our water is contaminated. I recommend that you purchase a good-quality water filter for your home, even if it's just for the kitchen tap. Don't drink from plastic bottles.

Dehydration can lead to memory loss, impaired cognition, and decreased mental performance. While the short-term effects of dehydration can be reversed by drinking water, chronic dehydration can have serious, long-lasting, negative effects on your brain. It's also important to note that your thirst receptors are not as precise as you age, so it's common for older people to get dehydrated.

The standard "rule" is eight 8-ounce glasses of water per day. But your physical activity, how much you sweat, the temperature and humidity levels of your environment, what you eat, the medications you take, and many other factors determine if that is enough.

Let your body tell you how much you need! When you're thirsty, drink. When you're not thirsty anymore, stop. If it's hot, you're exercising, or you're sweating, drink more.

I discussed the dangers of toxic water in great detail in chapter 7, so please revisit that chapter for ways to evaluate your water supply.

Healthy Fats

You can power your brain extremely efficiently with fat, creating more adenosine triphosphate (ATP) molecules and creating fewer damaging free radicals than when your brain is burning carbs. In fact, your brain does better using fat as a fuel as compared to glucose. (See chapter 14.)

Over the last 40 years people have been duped into believing that fat is bad for their health. That's obviously not the case – check out the current obesity rates compared to 40 years ago. But not all fats are equal, and there are many you should not consume. (See chapter 13.)

Where are the healthy fats?

Avocado Oil

Like the fruit itself, oil made from avocados is rich in monounsaturated fat, which decreases the bad cholesterol while increasing the good cholesterol.

...roves mitochondrial function,[27] and, ...eases oxidative stress in the brain.[28] ...reduce inflammation, and some re- ...ant source of CoQ10, which is es- ...rgy requirements – like the brain. ...uld use olive oil, and has a slightly ...d for roasting veggies. Buy pure, ...o oil, not an oil blend, though I ...ins its healing properties better

Coconut Oil

This is a somewhat controversial oil because of its high percentage of saturated fats. However, saturated fat is important as a component of cell membranes, including neurons. And coconut oil contains medium-chain triglycerides (MCT), which the liver metabolizes to ketone bodies, which are simple molecules that your cells can use as an alternative fuel. You can learn all about this process in chapter 14. A 2004 study showed that the administration of MCTs almost immediately improved cognitive function in older adults with memory disorders.[29] Another study showed that coconut oil reduced the amount of beta-amyloid plaques associated with this disease.[30]

Dr. Mary Newport recommends 20 gm of MCT oil per day, which is about two tablespoons of coconut oil.[31]

Olive Oil

Olive oil is a monounsaturated fat, and studies have shown that a higher intake of monounsaturated fats improves memory and other cognitive functions in seniors.[32] It also boosts levels of two important brain chemicals, brain-derived neurotrophic factor (BDNF)[33] and nerve growth factor (NGF).[34] It has high levels of vitamin E and polyphenols, which are potent antioxidants[35] and free-radical scavengers,[36] and it contains vitamin K, which has been shown to improve the ability to remember words.[37]

Olive oil helps protect against depression. An interesting study had participants replacing less healthy vegetable oils with olive oil, and their risk of depression plummeted by almost 50 percent.[38]

I use olive oil a lot, including for cooking if temperatures are not too high. But it's best used on salads, in mixtures like tahini, in marinades and sauces, and of course in pesto.

> *A word of caution: There are many "fake" oils out there labelled "extra virgin olive oil." They can contain canola or other unhealthy oils, and they can contain olive oil that has been processed or stored in dangerous conditions. Here you really do get what you pay for. Always buy the freshest extra virgin olive oil you can find, in dark glass bottles only. The older the oil is, the fewer polyphenols it contains due to oxidation.*

Sesame Oil

This tasty oil is rich in monounsaturated acids (MUFAs) and polyunsaturated acids (PUFAs) that cut cholesterol in the body. It is low in saturated fats while containing sesamol and sesamin, which are powerful antioxidants. It is also anti-inflammatory and helps with circulation.

Sesame oil has been used for centuries in holistic healing for its antibacterial, antiviral, and antifungal properties. It has a high smoke point, so it's good for cooking, especially stir-frying.

It's also beneficial when used topically and is often used as a carrier oil for essential oils.

> *A word of caution: Remember that* all *oils are high in calories, so if you are working to lose weight, you would do well to keep to a minimum the amount of oil you consume. For brain health, a non-fat diet is* not *recommended.*

Seeds

Many seeds are great sources of antioxidants – one of the many reasons they are so important for brain health. Your brain uses a lot of oxygen, so it's especially susceptible to free-radical attack – more than just about any other area of the body. And seeds have many other benefits.

Seeds contain a lot of fat, so many nutritionists and physicians recommend limiting the amount you eat. Like anything else, moderation is key, but throwing seeds on a salad and incorporating them in homemade, grain-free muffins or in smoothies are good ways to get the benefits of these powerful packages of nutrition.

Chia

These tiny seeds are full of omega-3 fatty acids, carbohydrates,[39] fiber, calcium, and antioxidants. They help keep your brain free from plaque and help brain cells communicate with one another. They can be baked into bread or muffins, and you can sprinkle them on just about anything. I include a great Chia Seed Pudding recipe in the appendix that also incorporates cinnamon, a powerful anti-inflammatory.

Hemp

Hemp hearts (hulled hemp seeds) are a balanced and rich source of both omega-6 and omega-3. They also contain gamma-linolenic acid, which helps with the growth and function of muscles, nerves, cells, and organs.

Hemp hearts have all the essential amino acids, so they are an excellent source of plant-based protein. Two to three tablespoons of hemp hearts provide about 11 grams of protein. They're also rich in calcium, iron, zinc, vitamin E, and other nutrients essential for heart health and to keep your arteries clean.

Whole hemp seeds contain both soluble and insoluble fiber, to support digestive and gut health.

Flax

Flax seeds are a rich source of fiber, omega-3 fatty acid,[40] alpha linolenic acid, and fiber. These compounds are anti-inflammatory, anti-oxidative, and help modulate lipids (fats and oils and hormones). These actions are essential for brain health, and a Japanese study has even shown that flax seeds worked better than antidepressants for treating depression. They are one of the few sources of omega-3 in a vegan diet, so be sure to eat them as often as you can.

Flax seeds soaked in water are a substitute for eggs in baking, and are delicious ground up for smoothies, in muffins, on salads, on peanut butter, in puddings, and many other ways.[41]

Pumpkin

Pumpkin seeds are concentrated sources of many nutrients, including the antioxidant vitamin E, minerals, antioxidants, and essential amino acids such as tryptophan and glutamate.[42] They have been shown to help increase quality of sleep, one of the most important things you must take care of to keep your brain healthy. They're a great snack on their own and add a terrific crunch to salads and another dimension to soups.

Sesame

These tasty seeds have been shown to have anti-inflammatory properties,[43] and this also extends to the oil from sesame seeds. Sesame seeds are easy to incorporate into your diet – on salads, in stir-fries, and as tahini mixed in a variety of foods including hummus.

Sunflower Seeds

Sunflower seeds are packed with fiber and are a great nutritional source of vitamins, especially vitamin E and selenium, both powerful antioxidants. They also contain vitamin B_6, which helps your body make norepinephrine and serotonin, which transmit brain signals.

Nuts

Nuts are very nutritious but, like seeds, they contain a lot of fat, so many nutritionists and physicians recommend limiting the amount you eat. Moderation is advisable, but the nuts below are simply too important nutritionally to avoid.

Almonds

There are many reasons almonds are good for the brain. Eating about two ounces of almonds daily for four weeks can help reduce insulin resistance, fasting insulin, and glucose. Since diabetes and insulin resistance are powerful drivers of dementia, that alone is reason enough to eat almonds.

Almonds have also been found to increase the levels of healthy bacteria in the gut,[44] and an ounce of almonds, which is about 25 almonds, contains

12 percent of our necessary daily protein. They are also rich in vitamin E; B vitamins; essential minerals like calcium, magnesium, and potassium; and healthy fat.

Brazil Nuts

These delicious nuts contain ellagic acid, which has been shown to have neu-roprotective properties.[45] Brazil nuts also contain large amounts of selenium, which is important in protecting against depression[46] and helps the immune system. For these reasons it makes good sense to add Brazil nuts to your list of potential snacking nuts, or to add them to your salads.

Cashews

Cashews are high in omega-3 fats, iron, magnesium, vitamin B_6, protein, and important amino acids like tryptophan. Studies have shown that these are all helpful in naturally warding off mild depression and anxiety.[47]

Tryptophan is critical for improving the uptake of serotonin, an antidepres-sant hormone, in the brain, and acts as a direct precursor to it.[48] Insufficient serotonin can make us feel anxious, stressed, and sad. The vitamin B_6 and tryptophan in cashews help with serotonin uptake, and the B_6 also helps all-important magnesium get to the cells more easily.

Cashews also contain magnesium and are among the best sources of mono-unsaturated fats. As a result, they help ward off depression naturally.

Coconuts

For the same reason that coconut oil is good for your brain, so are coco-nuts. Coconut water is great for hydration and electrolytes, and coconut flour contains more protein and fiber than wheat bran. Coconuts contain no added cholesterol (as animal foods do), and contribute to a healthy cholesterol level in the body. This is essential for brain health. Coconut meat, oil, and butter have amazing antibacterial and immune-boosting properties as well.

Coconut milk can be made into yogurt and ice "cream," and it's great on its own mixed with chia seeds and cinnamon for a pudding. The meat of the coconut is a delicious snack, and while it's readily available where I live in

Ecuador, it's more expensive and trickier to find in North America and Europe. But you can easily buy shaved coconut, which is great to sprinkle on granola and add to smoothies, and to make delicious muffins and quick breads. Make sure it's raw so all the nutrients remain intact.

Pecans

Pecans contain antioxidant phytonutrients and more flavonoids than any other tree nut. They are also an excellent source of vitamin E, which has been shown to reduce the risk of Alzheimer's disease and other dementias by up to 25 percent.

Pistachios

Like other nuts, pistachios are rich in antioxidants,[49] but they have a big advantage in that the antioxidants in pistachios are very *bioavailable*, meaning that they're more likely to be absorbed and used during the digestive process. Pistachios are rich in vitamin B_6, and you can get almost a whole day's worth, plus six grams of protein, in one small one-ounce serving. They are also high in vitamins A, K, and E. According to recent articles,[50] eating pistachios might increase the levels of beneficial bacteria in the gut.

Walnuts

I don't think it's a coincidence that walnuts look like little brains, because they are powerhouses that help protect your brain from dementia.

They are the only nuts that have a significant amount of alpha-linolenic acid (ALA), an essential omega-3 fatty acid. They also contain other polyphenols that act as antioxidants and appear to block the signals produced by free radicals that can cause or increase inflammation. Walnuts also nourish the beneficial bacteria in your gut and they contain serotonin, which is important for mood.

Walnut extract has been shown to inhibit the buildup of the beta-amyloid proteins[51] that are the hallmarks of Alzheimer's, and eating walnuts can improve reaction time, learning, and memory in adults of all ages.[52]

It doesn't take much – just one tablespoon a day can help improve cognitive health. I love walnuts as a snack and they are fantastic on fruit or vegetable salads. But one of my favorite ways to eat them is in vegan chocolate brownies, which also incorporate cacao and avocados. The recipe for this amazingly delicious and healthy dessert is in the appendix.

Legumes and Beans

In 2004 researchers from Japan, Sweden, Greece, and Australia teamed up to see if there was one food consumed by people in many cultures that could be linked to a longer lifespan. It turns out that the more beans, peas, soybeans, garbanzo beans (chickpeas), lentils, white beans, and even peanuts people ate, the longer they lived.

Legumes contain magnesium, potassium, folate, and iron, which can help with general body function and the firing of neurons. They also contain choline, a B vitamin that boosts acetylcholine, a neurotransmitter critical for brain function.

Grains and Substitutes

This group of foods is problematic because I believe the jury is still out on whether grains are harmful or beneficial for brain health. Dr. David Perlmutter claims they cause inflammation, which we know is a big contributor to dementia. In fact, in the next chapter called "Foods to Avoid and Why," I include the grains wheat, rye, barley, corn, millet, sorghum, spelt, and teff – especially if they are milled. However, there are some who have said that these grains can be beneficial if they are sprouted.

I believe the best course of action with grains is to err on the side of caution and eat only organic, sprouted grains in limited quantities. Organic wild and brown rice are not detrimental to your health in small quantities. But pay careful attention to how your body reacts when you eat these.

Quinoa

Quinoa botanically is not a grain, but the edible part – the seed – is often used as a grain. You generally see white quinoa at the store, but there are also red and black varieties. Black quinoa has the highest omega-3 fatty acid content, so it is best for brain health, but all have antioxidant properties. Quinoa is packed with vitamins and minerals including magnesium, manganese, iron, zinc, thiamin, riboflavin, and B$_6$, and is low in calories. One cup of cooked quinoa has only 220 calories but contains eight grams of protein and at least five grams of fiber.

The protein in quinoa is complete, meaning it contains all nine of the essential amino acids, important when your diet is plant-based. Quinoa is a great alternative to rice, is much more nutritious, and offers many more benefits to your brain. I include recipes in the appendix so that you can easily incorporate it into your diet.

Yucca, or Cassava

I know, putting a root in here seems crazy, but yucca is used more like a grain than a vegetable, so I'm placing it here because many people have never considered it as an alternative to grains. It comes from the cassava plant, which produces a starchy root from which we make yucca flour. It's gluten-free, grain-free, and nut-free; is low in calories, fat, and sugar; and is a great alternative to flour. It is also high in vitamin C.

Yucca flour is also known as cassava flour or tapioca flour in North America.[53] However, tapioca flour is more highly processed. It is extracted from the cassava plant through a process of washing and pulping. After extraction, the wet pulp is squeezed to create a starchy liquid. Once all the water evaporates, the tapioca flour remains. However, cassava or yucca flour is made simply from the ground-up root of the cassava plant with no other processes.

I learned of it here in Ecuador because it is one of the most valuable sources of nutrition for many people here and in Asia and Africa. It requires a low amount of energy to produce and yields a high amount of edible crop per plant, making it one of the world's most valuable, stable crops.

Its texture lends well to baking denser breads, or you can use it in savory dishes to thicken sauces or to form burgers/patties. It doesn't have a sour taste or smell like fermented, sprouted grain flours sometimes can.

There are a few recipes in the appendix utilizing this versatile food so you can see how delicious it can be.

Spices

Black Pepper

Who would ever have believed this humble kitchen staple could be so powerful? Black pepper has an active compound called piperine that increases beta-endorphins in the brain and boosts cognitive function. Beta-endorphins have neurotransmitter qualities that improve your mood and promote feelings of relaxation.

Turmeric

The active ingredient in turmeric is curcumin, which has a positive effect on gene expression.[54] That means that it can help prevent the Alzheimer's gene (and others) from being turned on. It does this partially through controlling the process of methylation, which is like an off/on switch that controls how genes express themselves.

Curcumin has also been shown to be beneficial in treating the symptoms of Crohn's disease, irritable bowel syndrome, and stomach ulcers. Since gut health is so incredibly important for brain health, this is an especially important spice to eat. It has also been shown to increase brain-derived neurotrophic factor (BDNF), which plays a key role in creating new neurons.

Curcumin also helps relieve arthritis pain and manage diabetes, heart disease, and a variety of autoimmune and inflammatory diseases like rheumatoid arthritis.

A common use of turmeric is in Golden Milk Turmeric Tea, which is used for pain and inflammation reduction. There are many videos describing how to make this on YouTube.

Adding a teaspoon of ground turmeric to smoothies is another great way to utilize this spice, but it is especially tasty in curries, stir-fries, soups, and stews. Many of the recipes in the appendix use this powerhouse.

Ginger

While we generally think of ginger as a root vegetable, it's considered a spice in the culinary world. If you're determined to improve the health of your brain, next to turmeric, ginger is probably one of the most important spices you can add to your diet. It boasts both anti-inflammatory and antioxidant activity. In several studies ginger was proved to be beneficial in lowering blood pressure, reducing inflammation, and acting as a neuro-protectant.[55] It has also been shown to lower fasting glucose levels, which is very important in controlling diabetes,[56] a primary cause of Alzheimer's.

Gingerol is the potent chemical in ginger and is what makes it decrease inflammation and maybe even block nerve pathways that process pain. Adding more ginger to your diet will help relieve pain and stiffness in knee joints,[57] which makes the all-important exercising easier and more fun.

The best way to consume it is raw and fresh. It adds pep to any smoothie or homemade salad dressing. It's also wonderful grated over salads and in oriental dishes. Steeped in hot water, it makes a soothing tea. Most studies use doses between one and two grams per day for adults.

Cardamom

This spice is less well known, but studies have shown it may be helpful in reducing blood pressure and protecting cells against damage. It acts as an anti-inflammatory. It is also known to squelch symptoms of upset stomach including nausea, heartburn, and irritable bowel syndrome, all symptoms of an unhealthy gut.

Chilies

Chili peppers are rich in vitamin A and they have been shown to reduce pain, fight free radicals, lower cholesterol, clear congestion, and boost immunity. Capsaicin is the powerful compound in chilies that has been shown to fight inflammation and get your blood flowing to the right places, including boosting circulation to benefit heart health.

Cinnamon

Cinnamon provides manganese, an important but often overlooked nutrient, and it has been shown to help prevent blood-sugar levels from spiking. It is also known for its anti-inflammatory, circulatory, and heart-strengthening properties.

A study published in the *Journal of Alzheimer's Disease* showed that the cinnamaldehyde and epicatechin in cinnamon inhibit the aggregation of tau proteins, which are serious components of Alzheimer's.

According to another study the compounds in cinnamon extract can help prevent brain cells from swelling,[58] thereby reducing complications related to traumatic brain injury and stroke, both of which can increase the likelihood of developing dementia.

Cinnamon also provides antioxidants that can protect against the free radicals that cause cognitive decline, and it can activate neuro-protective proteins that shield the cells of the brain, protecting them from damage.

It can easily be woven into sweet and savory dishes. Add it to everything you can! Sprinkle it in your coffee in the morning or make the Avocado-Banana Chocolate Pudding in the appendix.

Cumin

Cumin helps improve digestion by promoting the activity of digestive enzymes, and it is a good source of iron. As with other plant compounds, cumin's antioxidants help decrease inflammation and may be beneficial in helping control heart disease, diabetes, and cancer.

Vanilla

We don't often think of it as a medicinal spice, but vanilla is good for the brain. Vanilla bean powder contains magnesium, which optimizes neurotransmitter function for optimal serotonin and dopamine production and helps maintain healthy blood-sugar levels and blood pressure. It also contains calcium, which reduces the stress hormone cortisol. Manganese is also in vanilla bean powder, and one tablespoon has 30 percent of your daily manganese needs.

Vanilla beans and vanilla bean powder are the way to get all these benefits, not the extract. There is no set recommended amount – just use it as you would cacao for flavor.

Herbs

Oregano

Oregano has a high concentration of antioxidants. A study published in the *British Journal of Nutrition* found that the compounds in oregano inhibit the degradation of monoamine neurotransmitters, which are involved in modulating your mood, anxiety, cognition, sleep, and appetite. Oregano helps decrease anxiety and improve learning and concentration. It has also been shown in laboratory tests to have significant antibacterial activity, and in a meta-study researchers found that it appeared to have anti-inflammatory properties.[59] For treating and preventing type 2 diabetes, you can use oregano leaves and oil to improve insulin resistance.[60]

Use oregano in cooking, and the essential oil is great for relieving stress and calming your nerves. There has been some discussion about the possibility of using too much oregano oil because it can destroy good bacteria as well as the bad. So unless you are well-versed in the use of this as a therapeutic essential oil, it might be best to just ingest oregano in sauces, soups, and other dishes.

> *A word of caution: If you have allergic reactions to plants belonging to the mint family (which includes lavender), be cautious when using oregano.*

Psyllium Husk

Psyllium is a type of fiber, and most of us recognize it for its use as a laxative, which of course is important in keeping the intestinal tract healthy. But it has many more benefits. It has been shown to help patients who have type 2 diabetes control their blood sugar,[61] and to help with metabolic control.[62]

Adding psyllium husk and other water-soluble fibers to your diet helps lower your triglyceride levels and lower your risk of cardiovascular disease and hypertension, which helps lower the risk of vascular dementia. Psyllium has also been shown to help significantly decrease body weight, partially because it helps you feel full.

One way I use psyllium husk is to make Vegan Mozzarella and Vegan Butter. The recipes are in the appendix under "Vegan Basics."

Rosemary

Researchers have found that the antioxidants in rosemary can prevent age-related memory loss,[63] improve learning, and reduce oxidative damage in the brain. Rosemary is also known to inhibit neuronal cell death,[64] and it acts as an anti-inflammatory agent,[65] while rosemarinic acid has been shown to enhance cognition.

Seven hundred fifty mg per day of dried rosemary leaf powder seems optimal, but the study that confirmed this also advised that high doses of the herb can impair memory.[66] So as is the case with most things, more is not necessarily better.

Rosemary tea is one way to get a tasty dose every day. Put a small branch with leaves in a cup of boiling water and let it steep for 20 minutes, or leave it overnight. Strain and enjoy. And, of course, just add it as an herb to any savory dish.

Sage

Sage might help with chemical imbalances in the brain that cause symptoms of Alzheimer's disease, and studies suggest it improves how the body uses insulin and sugar. It also has anti-inflammatory properties.

During one study it was demonstrated that taking extracts of common sage and Spanish sage for four months improved learning, memory, and information-processing in people with mild to moderate Alzheimer's disease.[67] It's also been shown to enhance memory in both young and older volunteers with normal cognitive function.

Use as much as you like to spice things up.

For Your Sweet Tooth

Artificial sweeteners like aspartame and sucralose are obviously a big NO, (see chapter 13), but some other sweeteners can be used.

Maple syrup has several protective phytochemicals. It contains antioxidants, which help prevent cardiovascular disease, diabetes, and cancer. It also has a relatively low glycemic index, which helps in the prevention of type 2 diabetes. But most important for our purposes, there is evidence that it may help fight inflammation and neurodegenerative diseases. Its plant-based compounds reduce oxidative stress, which contributes to aging and brain-cell death. As with any other sweetener, use it in moderation.

Stevia, which is extracted from a plant of the same name, seems to have relatively few danger signals. While it seems to be benign toward your gut flora, like other sweeteners it might "fool" your body into thinking you have consumed sugar. This can trigger the same release of insulin, but because there is no additional glucose you might end up feeling more tired and, in fact, more desperate to consume other sources of actual sugar. On the balance of probabilities, it is probably okay to include it in your diet, but in moderation.

Xylitol is a sugar alcohol that comes from either birch tree bark or corn cob, but it is a lengthy industrial process to get it from the original source. It seems to be safe, and in fact beneficial in protecting teeth against plaque and cavities.[68] There is also some indication it can help protect against candida.[69] Another plus is that trials on human subjects showed that it does not raise blood glucose readings or have any impact on insulin levels.[70]

Some people do experience pain, bloating, and occasionally diarrhea from ingesting xylitol, but you need to have more than 50 grams at one time to get those effects. On the balance of probabilities, it is safer than many other sweeteners.

A word of caution: Xylitol is poisonous to pets, so you must be vigilant when you have animals in the house.

Erythritol, like xylitol, is a form of sugar alcohol. While it is also highly processed, this low-calorie sweetener has little to no effect on blood sugar and insulin levels. Some research showed that it may also feed the friendly bacteria in your gut. I have never used it, but it might be an alternative to xylitol since it's also safe for pets.

So there you have it – plenty of delicious, healthy foods to choose from in your brain-healthy lifestyle. In the next chapter you'll learn about foods that absolutely should be avoided.

Chapter 13

Foods to Avoid, and Why

Changing your lifestyle is not easy, especially when it comes to food. You have memories attached to food, and much of the food you get from restaurants and the middle aisles of grocery stores has been engineered to make you crave it. So I know this is a challenge.

But it will be worth it, and as you learn why some of your favorite foods might be threatening your brain and your long-term health, you should find it easier to keep your resolve to eat better.

Processed Food

Boxed macaroni and cheese. Canned sauces. Cookies and cupcakes. Boxed cereals. Besides creating insulin resistance and putting you at risk for diabetes thanks to the added sugar and/or artificial sweeteners, most processed foods are highly inflammatory because of the preservatives, refined flours and grains, artificial colorings and flavorings, and genetically modified ingredients.

Removing processed food from your diet also means avoiding many restaurants. Most big food chains source from factory farms; the food is not organic. And nearly everything at chain restaurants comes from a warehouse and is prepared with set amounts of sodium, preservatives, and the like.

It's hard to give up going out for dinner, though, and you don't have to. There is a trend toward "farm to table" restaurants where they work with local farmers to provide fresh, wholesome veggies, herbs, fruits, and grains like amaranth, right from local organic fields. Seek out these and other smaller restaurants. Yes, you will probably pay a bit more for your meal but – pay now or pay later.

Wheat and Most Grains

If grains are milled into flour, the starch in them has a high glycemic index. That means they convert rapidly into glucose, which causes a rise in blood sugar. Besides possibly triggering diabetes, this rise in blood sugar promotes the formation of advanced glycation end products (AGEs), which results in inflammation.[1]

Many grains are also contaminated with heavy metals like mercury, arsenic, and cadmium; molds and mycotoxins; and, of course, pesticides like glyphosate and atrazine.

Avoid wheat, rye, barley, corn, millet, sorghum, spelt, and teff. Some advocates say that rice and wild rice can be problematic for those with autoimmune diseases, but for the purposes of brain health, what I've learned is that as long as the rice you eat is organic and processed without possibility of gluten contamination, you can have it in moderation.

It's hard to eliminate oats because they have many benefits, including lowering cholesterol, and they are a good source of fiber. Unfortunately, oats are still grains, and even if you buy organic and are somehow lucky enough to find a brand that is not contaminated by wheat or other grains, there is some evidence that components in the oat proteins cause inflammation. That said, if you need to use a little as a binder in a recipe, that's fine. As I mentioned in chapter 12 – moderation is key.

Refined Carbohydrates and Sugar

If it's white, stay away: pasta, white rice, rice snacks, crackers, cakes, cookies and bagels, pastries, pizza dough, hamburger and hot dog buns, pancakes, and waffles. Anything that is highly refined is devoid of most nutrients and can spike blood sugar.

Instead of refined flours, opt for yucca or almond flour for baking, zucchini and carrot spirals instead of pasta, and quinoa instead of rice.

Dairy Products

Dairy products are notorious for causing inflammation (see chapter 3). Humans are the only mammals that consume milk beyond the breastfeeding years, and many scientists and nutritionists agree that we cease to produce the necessary enzymes to properly digest dairy products by the time we are eight years old.

There is also a protein in milk that leads to the production of a molecule that can cause an immune response, with symptoms such as skin reactions, rich mucus production, and inflammation. This molecule slows the passage of food through the digestive system, which causes its own inflammatory response and can trigger leaky gut.

Research shows that dairy intake reduces the abundance and the diversity of the gut microbiota, especially if you consume a lot of pasteurized milk products, which are essentially sterile in microbiota composition.

Industrial dairy products are high in dioxins, antibiotics, PCBs, and pesticides, wreaking havoc everywhere in your body.

This may be hard to believe if you're a big cheese fan, but once you eliminate it, you will never want to go back because you will feel so much better. I include easy recipes for delicious sunflower-seed-based Vegan Mozzarella and a creamy Vegan "Alfredo" Sauce that is much tastier than dairy-based Alfredo, with half the calories and triple the nutrients.

Meat and Poultry

Many diet and health gurus encourage you to eat the meat of free-range beef or turkey or chicken or pigs raised in "humane" conditions and "grass fed." I disagree. There is nothing humane about killing anything, and your brain is much better off without these products.

One study of more than 18,000 people found links between a diet high in fried food and processed meat and low scores in learning and memory.[2,3] Other research, which studied more than 5,000 people, found that a diet rich in red meat, processed meat, and fried food was associated with a faster decline in reasoning.[4]

Dr. Michael Greger, an expert in brain health, has pointed to evidence that in the U.S., those following a meat-free diet can cut their risk of developing dementia by more than half. When compared to people who eat meat more than four times a week, the dementia risk of people who have consumed vegetarian diets for 30 years or more is three times lower.

Even the 2014 "Dietary and Lifestyle Guidelines for the Prevention of Alzheimer's Disease" recommended swapping out animal products in favor of plant-based alternatives. "Vegetables, legumes [beans, peas, and lentils], fruits, and whole grains should replace meats and dairy products as primary staples of the diet." [5]

Alcohol

Consuming significant amounts of alcohol is obviously bad for you,[6] but there is increasing evidence that for brain health, it's not a good idea to ingest it at all.[7] This is partially because alcohol has the potential to skew the balance of good versus bad microbiota in the gut.[8] There is also some evidence to suggest that it can contribute to leaky gut syndrome.

That said, however, other studies have shown that moderate consumption (one to six glasses per week) of red wine may have beneficial effects and can lower the risk of dementia among older adults.[9]

For safety's sake, if you're serious about preventing dementia, it's probably better to err on the side of caution and forego the alcohol. But don't beat yourself up if you have a glass of red wine at your niece's wedding!

Soft Drinks

Sugar-filled soft drinks are harmful in so many ways, it could take a whole book just to describe what they do to you. The high quantity of sugar alone is enough to put this on the "avoid list," but in the case of colas, you also have phosphoric acid, which acidifies your body. If it can remove rust, you really don't want to drink it.

Many soft drinks also contain artificial sweeteners. See more about them below.

Aspartame, Sucralose, and All Artificial Sweeteners

Contrary to what we've been told by the industry that sells them, artificial sweeteners are poison. They change the microbiome in a way that not only paves the way to obesity, but also to type 2 diabetes. The evidence is overwhelming that the very foods people are eating in hopes of getting rid of that big belly are having the exact opposite effect, and in the process they are putting their brains at risk.

Aspartame is 40 percent aspartic acid, which functions as an excitotoxin, stimulating neurons and destroying nerve cells. That's the last thing you need when you're trying to save your brain.

These artificial sweeteners are snuck into many products these days, so you must read labels *very* carefully. I've seen sucralose in everything from liquid vitamins to protein powders, and of course aspartame is in gum and many other products.

Vegetable Oils and Trans Fats

Vegetable and seed oils are often extracted from the seeds of plants using harsh solvents like hexane, which is a component of gasoline. This includes oils like soybean, corn, peanut, safflower, sunflower, and canola (also known as rapeseed).

One research team found that soybean oil induces diabetes and obesity in mice, and it has a major impact on their hypothalamus,[10] an area of the brain crucial for regulating mood and behavior. It also affected over 100 of the mice's genes, including one for controlling oxytocin, the love and bonding hormone.

Artificial trans fats are normally listed as "partially hydrogenated" oil in the ingredients lists of processed foods like crackers, frozen foods, and margarine. They're added to extend shelf life. They cause inflammation and increase the risk of all diseases.[11]

When foods fried in hydrogenated oils are heated to extreme temperatures (think French fries and potato chips), they can release advanced glycation end products, which are chemicals that are also released when meat and dairy products are heated.

Canola oil is another oil to stay away from. It is touted as a healthy oil because it is low in erucic acid, high in oleic acid (just like heart-healthy olive oil), high in omega-3 fats, and it's neutral-tasting. There are many problems with this oil, though, not the least of which is genetic modification, which is problem enough, but that also means it is sprayed with copious amounts of glyphosate.

A study out of Temple University and published in the journal *Scientific Reports* linked canola oil with higher amounts of amyloid plaques as well as diminished contact between brain neurons.[12] This leads to a decrease in memory and learning.

Margarine. There are so many things wrong with this poison I barely know where to start, but I'll address diacetyl, one of its ingredients. This has been shown to promote the clumping of beta-amyloid, one of the proteins implicated in Alzheimer's. It is also suspected of reducing glyoxalase I, which is one of the body's primary response factors in detoxifying amyloid in the brain.

Stick to coconut oil; 100 percent pure, cold-pressed, organic olive oil; and avocado oil.

Monosodium Glutamate (MSG)

Often found in chain-restaurant food and Chinese food, MSG can be deadly for some people, and it is simply not good for anyone's brain. There is a pretty strong lobby out there trying to convince us that it is safe, but a powerful report from 1995 concludes, in part: "MSG causes brain damage, learning disorders, obesity, stunted growth, infertility, and other endocrine problems."[13] Avoid it like the plague.

Anything That Contains Genetically Modified Organisms (GMO) or Is Treated with Glyphosate

I've covered this in many ways, including in chapter 7 about toxins, and throughout with respect to inflammation. I know it is almost impossible to avoid glyphosate[14] and many other pesticides and herbicides because they have literally polluted the planet, but do your best. Eat organic if possible.

&

It's mostly common sense when it comes to avoiding foods that are bad for your brain because most of them have been "outed" because they cause cancer, hypertension, and a myriad of other problems. By eating to save your brain, you're also protecting yourself against these other diseases.

Chapter 14

Fasting, Autophagy, and Ketosis

One of the best things you can do for your brain is to fast, or more accurately, practice time-restricted eating. I won't get into all the processes that make fasting work – that is the subject of a whole book, and there are experts out there who do an excellent job of explaining it. Dr. David Jockers is one, and I recommend that if you're interested in learning more, you should check out his work.[1]

Fasting is important because it allows your body to clean out the debris after it has processed the food you have given it. If you stop eating for six hours or more, your body gets into a cleansing phase in which it tears down old, damaged cells. This process turns on genetic repair mechanisms through the release of human growth hormone (HGH).

HGH changes your metabolism to favor fat-burning and to save proteins so that they and amino acids can be used to improve brain and neuron processing. Research has shown this state helps boost good (HDL) cholesterol and reduce inflammation,[2] which, as you've learned, is a huge contributor to dementia.

Intermittent fasting also helps resolve insulin resistance.[3] Since elevated levels of circulating insulin cause metabolic problems as well as accelerated degenerative states, this alone would be a good reason for intermittent fasting. A 2014 study found that intermittent fasting lowered blood sugar by 3 to 6 percent and fasting insulin levels by 20 to 31 percent. At the same time it forces your brain to use ketones as a fuel. These are a much cleaner and more efficient fuel than carbohydrates.

According to Dr. Mark Mattson, a professor of neurology at Johns Hopkins University, fasting increases the rate of neurogenesis in the brain.[4] That means you're building more new brain cells.

Limiting the time you eat and the size of your meals also boosts production of brain-derived neurotrophic factor (BDNF),[5] which helps produce new brain cells, protect the brain cells you have, and stimulate new connections and synapses. All this while also boosting memory and improving mood and learning. Low levels of BDNF have been linked to dementia, memory loss, and other brain processing problems.[6]

When you combine fasting and exercise, you put the body in a healthy state of stress, which propels it into a building phase. This helps enhance connections between neurons and improves brain function.

To make fasting as easy and effective as possible, you should prepare your body for it. It would be difficult to go from eating all day to eating only eight hours in the day! That's why I stress removing sugar (yes, all of it) and processed carbohydrates from your diet early in the Eight Weeks to a Better Brain program. It's important to balance your blood sugar and regulate your insulin as much as possible before undertaking time-restricted eating. *If you have any problems with diabetes or insulin resistance, do not do this without consulting your doctor!*

By eating a whole-foods, plant-based diet that includes good fats like those in coconuts and coconut oil, olives and olive oil, avocados and avocado oil, and nuts for at least a week, you will be ready to begin intermittent or time-restricted fasting.

In this program the goal is to build up to eating during only eight hours a day. This is not going to happen all at once. You'll start with a 12-hour fast two days per week. That means you stop eating after dinner and don't eat again until at least 12 hours later, for breakfast. It's actually pretty easy because you're sleeping eight of those hours. Many people can go 14 hours or more without even thinking about it because their body is not starving for the sugars they've eliminated.

Once your body is used to this, you can do a 12- to 14-hour fast four or five days a week, or extend it to 16 hours a day. Mostly that's what we do at our house – every day includes at least a 12-hour fast, but many days it's 16 hours between the last meal of the day before and "lunch" the next day. It's not difficult, and I say this as someone who was hypoglycemic most of my adult life.

If you are generally healthy, just by doing intermittent fasting and changing your diet to whole foods with no processed carbohydrates you should see some weight loss as well as an improvement in your brain function. Brain fog should start to diminish and memory for things like names and appointments could improve. Part of the reason for this is because your brain is getting rid of the rubbish that it accumulates. This is called *autophagy*, which is an important part of improving brain function.

What Is Autophagy?

Autophagy is a natural process that recycles or removes unwanted molecules and dysfunctional parts of cells. Brain autophagy removes old and damaged brain cells so that new and healthy ones can be created. This process is essential for memory, cognition, and brain health, and it helps reduce brain degeneration.

Autophagy comes about in part from "stressful" processes like nutrient deprivation brought on from things like fasting (whether it's intermittent or for extended periods), exercise, and significant temperature change.

Because autophagy cleans out toxins and other infectious agents, it also plays an essential role in the immune system and in controlling inflammation,[7] which we know is important for brain health.

How to instigate autophagy? Fasting and simple caloric restriction alone can be effective, but if you combine the two, it is even more efficient.[8] Exercise also puts the cells under stress because it damages and inflames some cell components. The authors of one paper explained that our cells respond to this stress by instigating autophagy.[9]

It's been found that curcumin (which is found in turmeric) can induce autophagy in people who have diabetes,[10] and a study in mice suggested that curcumin can help fight cognitive impairment due to chemotherapy by inducing autophagy in certain regions in the brain.[11]

Hot and cold therapy can also help clean up old cells. You will learn more about that in chapter 19 about alternative therapies.

Another way to clean up these old and damaged cells is to get into a state of *ketosis*. Keto diets are extremely popular now, so let's understand what this really means, and how ketosis affects the brain.

What Do Ketones Have to Do with the Brain?

Our brains normally run on glucose (sugar). This is especially true now, when so many people are ingesting the standard American diet (SAD), or what I call the "standard Alzheimer's diet." This works fine when we are younger, but as we age it is harder to get glucose into our brains, thanks in part to insulin resistance. After age 40 or so, not only do our brains have more of a challenge running on glucose, but our metabolism changes as well, which is one of the reasons we gain weight as we age.

For our brains to run on this glucose, insulin must get into the cells. Glucose transporters from the insulin allow the glucose to get into the brain through the blood/brain barrier. But if the transporters don't work, the neurons can't get the glucose, so they begin to die. That's why the symptoms of cognitive decline and dementia begin to manifest. That's also why some people call Alzheimer's disease "type 3 diabetes." Just as with diabetes, the cause of insulin resistance in the brain isn't known, but it could very well be from excessive sugar and processed carbohydrates in the diet.

It's fortunate that our brains are wired to operate on other nutrients besides glucose; and we can set them up for an alternate fuel source – ketones. Since our ancestors couldn't always find or kill food, the human body adapted to be able to withstand periods of famine (fasting).

After 36 to 48 hours, we use up all the glucose in our bodies. Once it's gone, the fuel source switches and fat is converted in the liver to fatty acids, which the heart, muscles, and other organs use. However, these fatty acids can't cross the blood-brain barrier, so the liver converts some of the fat into ketone bodies.

Ketones are tiny, and enter the same biochemical path as glucose, but they do not require insulin to get into the cell. Once there, they make the final energy molecule the brain uses to fuel the cells.

This is one reason keto diets work so well for weight loss. The lack of carbohydrates and glucose means the body uses the stored fat.

However, that's not the only way to get those ketones. Coconut oil and the medium-chain triglyceride (MCT) oils that are in coconut oil can take the place of your body's fat. MCT is a healthy type of saturated fatty acid that has been linked to several important health benefits including improved cognitive function and support with weight management. MCT oils don't require digestives enzymes, so they are absorbed and go directly into the liver.

Some of the MCTs are converted to ketones; the rest are released and used immediately as energy. They are not stored as fat. These ketones can then cross the blood-brain barrier and feed the brain cells.

So you can achieve a state of ketosis by using MCTs and/or coconut oil as an alternative fuel to glucose. Since aging brains don't process glucose well, this is an excellent way to help with neurogenesis.

I can almost hear you saying, "But coconut oil is saturated fat!" Yes, 62 to 65 percent of coconut oil is in the form of MCTs, so let's address this issue of fats and the diet right now, because it will come up as you begin preparing the meals for this program.

The Fat Scare

It was the "no fat/low fat" diet fad that sent the Western world into carbohydrate overdrive. Dr. Ancel Keyes was the instigator. He took data from 22 countries in the world and looked at the level of fat in the diet and heart disease, correlating those areas where there was more fat in the diet to a higher incidence of heart disease. Makes sense, right?

However, he did not use the data from all countries. He only put nine of the points on his graph, which made it look like the more fat in the diet, the more heart problems. However, if you plot all the data that was available on a graph, the results are random.[12] There is no firm correlation between fat consumption and heart disease.

Unfortunately, the "science" Keyes presented propelled Western civilization into a tailspin of diabetes and obesity that is the result of too many carbohydrates, particularly those from processed foods. He did not espouse eating all the refined carbohydrates that are in the modern diet, but when you eliminate fat, taste and calories have to come from something else, and Big Food was right there waiting to fill the gap.

It's important to remember, though, that just because the no fat craze turned out to be based on false premises, it does not mean you should haphazardly add fats back into your diet. There is a big difference between good and bad fats, and you can't add even the good fats like coconut oil to your diet and not expect to gain weight if you don't take out other sources of calories. In this program you do that by getting rid of simple carbohydrates and dairy products and loading up on vegetables.

I digressed a bit, but I think it's important to understand the fat issue. For our purposes, the takeaway is that MCT oil can help keep ketones at a steady level over the course of a day. The goal is to ultimately help your brain function better, and you can do that by giving it this alternative fuel source.

There are three basic ways to achieve a state of ketosis:

1. Through intermittent fasting you can get into a state of ketosis daily, and while it is not sustained through the day, it does help
2. By eating a low-carbohydrate, high-fat, medium-protein diet – this is a lot of work and you must count every carbohydrate, but it's the basis of the keto diet
3. By adding MCT oil and coconut oil to your diet

What's the best approach? I believe that a combination of these makes the most sense. Fast at least 12, preferably 16 hours a day and eat a whole-foods, plant-based diet that is low in carbs and high in healthy fats, including coconut and MCT oil. Easy and delicious. There are several tasty recipes using coconut oil in the appendix.

જી

Of course, whenever you're changing your diet, or restricting it in any way, you must be sure to supply your body with the nutrients it needs. Up next, we'll look at the nutrients essential for a healthy brain and ways to ensure you're getting everything you need.

Chapter 15

Nutrition and Dementia

Our bodies are designed to operate perfectly with vitamins, minerals, and other nutrients that exist naturally in our food. Perhaps I should rather say, that *should* exist naturally in our food. Unfortunately, as we discussed in chapter 3, the soil is not what it used to be, and our bodies are stressed by unnatural compounds in our environment. Thus we have a bit more of a challenge getting optimal nutrition for our general health and our brains.

Because of these challenges, I want to address how and where you can get the nutrients that are most intimately connected to brain health, and discuss ways you can supplement if you find you are deficient in any of them.

Vitamins

B Vitamins

B vitamins are known for their stress-reduction properties, which alone is important for brain function. They can also halt memory loss and ward off brain aging.

The B vitamins, including folic acid, B_6, and B_{12}, all help prevent the atrophy of grey matter. A study at Oxford University showed that supplementation of B complex containing 800 micrograms (mcg) of folic acid, 20 mg of B_6, and 500 mcg of B_{12} reduced the loss of neurons in patients with mild cognitive decline.[1]

Sources of B vitamins include fruits, legumes, seeds, vegetables, and whole grains, so eating a whole-foods, plant-based diet means you get plenty of most of the B vitamins you need from your food.

There is one B vitamin that is particularly difficult to get no matter what your diet. Vitamin B$_{12}$ comes from a bacterium in the soil, and when you ingest it, it helps build the vitamin in the gut and regulates red blood cell function to prevent anemia. Unfortunately, the soil has been so depleted that this bacterium isn't available to feed your gut. This is why most people should take a supplement.

Up to 62 percent of adults over the age of 65 have less than optimal blood levels of vitamin B$_{12}$ even though the recommended daily allowance (RDA) is only 2.4 mcg. One study among many has shown that because the absorption rate is so low, you may need to supplement with 500 mcg of vitamin B$_{12}$, and for some people who are very active or under a lot of stress, 2,500 mcg may be necessary. It is a good idea to get checked for this nutrient.

Vitamin C

Several studies over many years show that Vitamin C is crucial for the brain's operation.[2] In fact, when your body starts to run out of vitamin C, it will vanish from every other organ before your body will allow its removal from your brain.

You must have adequate vitamin C throughout your life, because it doesn't do any good to supplement after you have already begun to exhibit symptoms of dementia.

How much to take? As is the case with most vitamins, the U.S. government's RDA for vitamin C is lower than many experts recommend – just 90 mg for men and 75 mg for women. That is just too low to keep your brain well-supplied. This vital antioxidant helps protect every part of your body, so you must have adequate amounts. I recommend 2,000 mg per day in supplement form. You should also aim to get vitamin C from foods including kale, kiwi, lemons, papaya, guava, oranges, strawberries, Brussels sprouts, and broccoli. Vitamin C is water soluble, so you can't really "overdose." People can sometimes get an upset stomach if they orally take more than 10,000 mg a day.

Vitamin D$_3$

Many people in North America are deficient in this vitamin, and a lack of it has been definitively linked to many health issues including Alzheimer's and other dementias.[3] Certainly deficiency in this vitamin has a link to thyroid issues,[4] which in turn lead to autoimmune diseases and depression, which in turn can lead to dementia. Deficiency of vitamin D$_3$ can also contribute to the danger of stroke,[5] which often leads to vascular dementia.

In the U.S., current guidelines suggest consuming 400 to 800 international units (IU) (10 to 20 mcg) of vitamin D$_3$, but several papers have been released[6] indicating that the lowest recommended dietary intake for adults should be at least 800 IU per day (IU/d), and doses up to at least 2,000 IU/d should be considered safe.

Unless you spend a lot of time outside and can manufacture your own vitamin D through exposure to the sun, you should probably take a supplement.

Vitamin E

As you probably expect, none of the vitamins and minerals you need to run your body and brain work in a vacuum. They need each other to ensure that everything runs smoothly. For brain health, the interaction of two vitamins has spurred a fair amount of research. Two studies involving more than 6,000 people found that vitamin E together with vitamin C produced a "lower risk of Alzheimer's disease."[7]

A Chicago study followed 815 adults 65 and older for four years and found that those who consumed the largest amount of vitamin E-rich foods, including leafy green vegetables, nuts, and whole grains, lowered their risk of developing Alzheimer's by 70 percent. Unfortunately, they also found that vitamin E alone did not positively affect those who carried the APOE4 gene. However, a Dutch study looked at 5,395 people 55 and older for six years and concluded that a diet high in both vitamins E and C lowered Alzheimer's risk even when the gene was present.

Decline in verbal fluency has been noted as an early predictor of the development of dementia. This was the basis of a study that showed that verbal fluency scores were consistently higher in test subjects who took vitamins E and C or vitamin E alone.[8]

On its own, vitamin E helps reduce oxidative stress caused by inflammation; but it isn't just a preventive. Research published in *The New England Journal of Medicine* showed that vitamin E supplements can impede the progression of Alzheimer's. Some doctors prescribe high doses to slow down the disease when no other treatments exist or have proven useful.

It's easy to get vitamin E from your diet. Nuts, sunflower seeds, peanuts, hazelnuts, pecans, spinach, broccoli, kiwi, mangoes, and asparagus are just a few of the delicious sources of vitamin E. The RDA for adults is 15 mg per day. If you decide you need to supplement, be sure to get the naturally sourced vitamin E: *d-alpha-tocopherol*.

Vitamin K

Vitamin K is a group of fat-soluble vitamins that share similar chemical structures.

Research indicates the higher one's vitamin K levels, the better their consolidation of memories. It has also been found that when geriatric patients were taking pharmaceuticals that depleted their levels of vitamin K, their executive function declined much more rapidly than that of patients who did not take these drugs (warfarin, acenocoumarol, and fluindione). [9]

Vitamin K in all its forms is important for synthesizing essential fats (think omega-3) in the brain, so this could be why it promotes healthy cognitive function and may prevent the development of dementia. It has also been shown to reduce the risk of diabetes by improving insulin function and decreasing insulin resistance.

K_1 is abundant in green beans and peas and in leafy green vegetables like spinach, kale, collard greens, turnip greens, and beet greens. K_2 sources vary. It is found in fermented foods and animal products but is also produced by gut bacteria.

If you are eating a whole-foods, plant-based diet with fermented foods as recommended in the Eight Weeks to a Better Brain program, you should be getting all you need.

If you do feel you need to take a supplement, be sure it contains both K_1 and K_2.

Minerals

Calcium

The nervous system needs calcium in order to operate properly, so mood issues, depression, and anxiety often result from a deficiency. Since depression especially is a known factor in developing dementia, it is important to address it right away.

On the other hand, a new study appeared to confirm a link between calcium supplements and an increased risk of dementia in older women who have had strokes.[10] So the recommendation is that such women not take any calcium supplements. It's better to get your calcium from foods anyway, including soy products and tofu (as long as they are non-GMO), almonds, oatmeal, and green vegetables.

The RDA is 1,000 mg for most adults, though women over 50 and everyone over 70 should get 1,200 mg per day.

Magnesium

Magnesium plays a part in more than 300 of the body's biochemical reactions, but thanks to our depleted soil, modern farming techniques, and less-than-ideal diets, most people do not get enough to protect their brains. And as we age it is more difficult to maintain magnesium levels in the cells, so magnesium deficiency is a big problem.

Researchers took a close look at more than 6,000 women between the ages of 65 and 79 and the amount of magnesium they were consuming. Those who got between about 257 and 317 mg per day had a significantly lower risk of developing cognitive impairment compared to the individuals who got only 197 mg or less per day.[11]

Magnesium also improves brain plasticity, something I discuss further in chapter 16. A Chinese study showed that increasing the level of magnesium helped nourish and energize brain cells, which resulted in less memory loss and other forms of age-related cognitive decline.[12]

A low magnesium level is also connected to vitamin D_3 deficiency. As discussed above, vitamin D_3 is important for your brain, so this is another reason to be sure you're getting enough magnesium.

As is the case with most nutrients, the RDA is incredibly low, only 420 mg per day for men and 320 mg per day for women, but most North Americans don't even get that much. The average intake of magnesium ranges between 143 and 266 mg per day.

The best way to get magnesium is from your food, of course: spinach, Swiss chard, and nuts like Brazil nuts, almonds, and cashews. Squash and pumpkin seeds and dark chocolate are also great sources, but pure cacao is healthier than chocolate. Add it to a smoothie or your coffee. Eating these foods also provides other much-needed minerals and vitamins.

Because of the contamination of our soil, many people require magnesium supplementation even if they are following a brain-healthy diet. Many nutritionists, including myself, recommend up to 1,000 mg per day for optimum brain health.

Potassium

People who are deficient in potassium often suffer from memory loss and confusion because the neurons in the brain rely on electrical signals generated by sodium and potassium channels in each neuron. Potassium deficiency can also impact your ability to learn.

Oxidative damage leads to decreased brain function, but potassium helps scavenge free radicals to counteract oxidation and prevent brain damage.

The National Institutes of Health recommends getting 4.7 grams of potassium per day, and it's easy to get enough by eating fresh fruits, dark leafy greens, coconut water and coconut oil, spinach, sweet potatoes, Brussels sprouts, and bananas. If you're following the whole-foods, plant-based diet in this book, you won't have to worry about potassium deficiencies.

Zinc

Zinc is essential for the healthy functioning of the body, including the brain. But many older people do not consume enough zinc, and even if they do, they are unable to absorb much of what they do consume.

Zinc is essential for dealing with stress and is required to synthesize the calming neurotransmitter GABA discussed in chapter 8.[13] Thus it is especially important for prevention of depression.

Zinc's role in the brain is essentially to reduce inflammation, and researchers have found that low levels of zinc can make inflammation in the brain worse. That can directly impact the progression of Alzheimer's in someone who already has the disease. On the other hand there are some studies indicating that excess zinc might be a factor in the development of dementia. To play it safe, it is best not to take a zinc supplement if you are getting sufficient zinc in your diet.

The recommended dose is 30 to 40 mg per day of zinc to help improve brain function in people with dementia. For healthy individuals without dementia, the RDA is 8 mg for women and 11 mg for men.

Plant foods high in zinc include pumpkin and hemp seeds, garbanzo beans (chickpeas), lentils, cocoa powder, mushrooms, spinach, avocados, almonds, and cashews.

Other Nutrients

Coenzyme Q_{10}

Coenzyme Q_{10} (CoQ10) is present in every cell in the body. CoQ10 functions in the mitochondria, so diseases like Alzheimer's, which are characterized by dysfunction of the mitochondria due to the aging process, are improved by taking a supplement of this compound.

There has been quite a bit of research on it, but the most impressive was a study published in the journal *Atherosclerosis*. It revealed that higher levels of CoQ10 in the blood correlate with a lowered risk of dementia in the later years of life.[14]

Oxidative stress is another aspect of aging that results in inflammation, particularly of the brain. However, studies are emerging that show that supplementing with CoQ10 helps prevent the neurodegeneration brought about by oxidative stress.[15]

A CoQ10 supplement would be helpful for most people as it is difficult to get enough in a standard diet. This compound has shown very few adverse effects even when people used up to 3,000 mg per day in clinical trials. The standard daily dose is 100 to 500 mg, with the highest recommended dosage at 1,200 mg per day.

Gingko Biloba

You've probably seen gingko biloba (gingko) being marketed for brain health. The supplements generally contain extracts of the plant's leaves, although the seeds are used for healing purposes in traditional Chinese medicine.

Ginkgo contains numerous flavonoids, and thus acts as an antioxidant and improves blood flow to the brain. Some studies have shown that in healthy people it can help boost memory and cognitive speed, although the results are far from conclusive. Several studies have shown that it can help with memory problems caused by dementia by preventing, for a time, the progression of symptoms, especially if the dementia is caused by vascular disease.

However, it can sometimes cause side effects such as allergic skin reactions, diarrhea, digestive problems, dizziness, headaches, muscle weakness, and nausea. So while it could be of value, it's not something I include in the Eight Weeks to a Better Brain program or in the protocols I recommend for my clients who are otherwise healthy and just want to protect their brains.

There is no RDA for gingko, but a common dose for people who have dementia is 40 mg of the extract three times daily. To study improving cognitive function in healthy people, researchers have used between 120 and 600 mg daily.

Omega-3 Fatty Acids

DHA and EPA are omega-3 fatty acids. These polyunsaturated fats have been related to a reduced risk for dementia.

DHA is an essential component of the cerebral cortex,[16] the area of the brain responsible for memory, language, abstraction, creativity, judgment, emotion, and attention. DHA also assists in the production of the important neurotransmitters dopamine, GABA, acetylcholine, and serotonin, all of which are essential to a healthy brain. It is such a crucial building block that people with low levels of it actually have measurably smaller brains![17]

To decrease the risk of dementia,[18] especially among those who do not have the APOE4 gene – it's important to include omega-3-rich oils along with lots of fruits and vegetables. Healthy adults should aim for between 250 and 2,000 mg of omega-3 daily. On the plant-based Eight Weeks to a Better Brain program, the best place to get it is from flax seeds, seaweed, and algae. Chia seeds, hemp seeds, and walnuts also contain them. You can also buy vegan supplements made from farm-raised, organic algae oil, which is recommended to ensure you're not getting mercury or other contaminants from the ocean with your omega-3.

There is no official recommendation for how much EPA and DHA are required, but Dr. David Perlmutter recommends that you get at least 1,000 mg of DHA per day.[19]

> *If you're on blood thinners or other medication, be sure to talk to your doctor before supplementing with omega-3.*

This list is by no means meant to be comprehensive of all the nutrients you need. These are considered especially important for brain health, and deficiencies are common. If you think you might be suffering from any kind of nutritional deficiency, I advise you have a full workup done by your integrative practitioner or physician.

Chapter 16

Exercise Your Body and Mind to Grow Your Brain

Move Your Body

As I pointed out in chapter 6, the single best thing you can do to help prevent dementia is to get moving. There is just no denying the positive impact that exercise has on the brain. If you need to go back and read the research about and reasons to exercise presented in chapter 6, please do so.

It's a challenge if you've been sedentary most of your life, but this is non-negotiable. You must move, especially to get your heart pumping. Cardiovascular exercise feeds and strengthens the blood vessels in your brain.

Here are some simple ways to move your body:

1. **Walk – preferably outside:** For a start, move as fast as you can at a pace that elevates your heart rate but still allows you to hold a conversation.

   Add some music to your walk. Brisk walking is 100 paces per minute. That will get your heart pumping, so play music that inspires you to move at that pace.

2. **Dance:** I cover more about dancing in chapter 18, but whenever you can, wherever you can – *dance!* Besides the physical benefits, it's also good for your mood.

3. **Weight training:** The benefits of strength and resistance training are especially important as you age. Not only do they protect against bone loss, they also help improve cognitive function. The stronger you get, the greater the benefit for your brain.

4. **Yoga, qigong, and tai chi:** Not only are these practices excellent for stress reduction and settling your mind, they can be started very gently with something like chair yoga. As you improve your health with all the good food you're eating on this program, you will be able to do more and your practice will evolve beyond gentle stretching to strength training and more.

There are countless videos online, but if you can, join a live class. Practicing this way gives you the benefit of being with others who are also working not just to improve their bodies but also their minds, and to connect with their spiritual sides. (See more about this in chapter 20.)

It is essential that your exercise be consistent, so aim for doing it at least a half hour a day. If you have any preexisting conditions or are completely out of shape, consult a physician before beginning or changing your workout routine.

Exercise Your Mind

We used to believe that once we got past 30 years old our brains started to die – the cells died off naturally or we killed them off by drinking alcohol, smoking pot, or living in a polluted environment. While it's true that these things can have negative effects on our brains, the good news is that our brains can not only continue to learn and change as we age, they can grow.

The human brain is not limited to the number of neurons it is born with, nor even to the additional neurons that fill in after the explosion of brain development in early childhood. Our brains can generate new neurons and neurons can adapt and change in response to stimuli. New pathways for the dissemination of energy and information can grow and strengthen.

Neurogenesis

Neurogenesis refers to the generation of new neurons from stem cells.[1] It's important in embryos and during early development, but it doesn't stop there. In adults, neurogenesis can occur in the hippocampus region of the brain where learning, memory, and emotions are processed. When our environment stimulates us, our mental energy increases, which can help diversify the development of new neural cells.

Neuroplasticity

We've heard a lot about this in the last few years… that our brains are plastic; that they change. But what does that mean?

Neuroplasticity involves learning.[2] When we are learning something, we inspire change in the brain. First, chemical changes occur. For example, when you're learning a language, you learn new vocabulary and remember it that day because that activity of learning those words has resulted in your brain changing chemically. But chemical changes are only good for short-term memory.

Next, to make that learning stick, and for it to stay in long-term memory, your brain needs to change structurally. It physically changes with practice as you work on this new learning. Those words you learned must be practiced and used in context so that your brain structurally changes to accommodate that information.

In the final step, functional changes occur. This involves making new connections between neurons and strengthening existing synapses. Let's go back to the language example:

You learn a new word or phrase on one day, but it is only a chemical change, so it's just there in your short-term memory. To be able to pull upon that new learning, you must practice by integrating that new vocabulary into your everyday speech. That changes the way the signals get around your brain. That is the structural change. Those words or phrases will now be there, but you will have to translate. The final step is when new connections have been made, and the way the neurons fire is functionally changed. Now the new language is integrated into your neural network and you begin to think in that new language. The brain has chemically, structurally, and functionally changed. That is neuroplasticity.

But there's a warning here. Neuroplasticity can be positive, but it can also be negative. If you start thinking negatively, lose your temper, or become addicted to drugs, that behavior also changes your brain, but for the worse. That's why it is so hard to overcome addictions, negative thinking, and the like.

What does this have to do with protecting against dementia? By making the brain change – by giving it chemical, structural, and functional challenges – it can become protected against the ravages of time and lifestyle. By using the wonderful gift of (positive) neuroplasticity, you are protecting your brain from negative changes.

But this is not something that happens just by playing computer games. It involves practice, and the harder something is the more it changes your brain and the more protection you have. This is why those of us working with people to protect their brains against dementia recommend learning a new language, learning to play a musical instrument, or acquiring a new motor skill like salsa dancing, skating, painting, or knitting.

It's not just the number of brain cells you have and if you can grow new ones; what is more important is how your brain uses the cells and creates new highways for information.

Let's do a quick check:

Are You Helping Your Brain Grow?

1. How often do you travel, especially to places that are different from your normal environment?
2. Do you go to the same restaurants all the time or do you like to try different foods?
3. Have you taken any community college or online courses lately?
4. Do you volunteer?
5. Have you studied or do you know a second language?

If you're stuck in a routine, or haven't actively learned anything for many years, now is a good time to get out of the rut. While physical activity alone can help induce neuroplastic changes in brain structure and function, it's not enough to save your brain. Choose a couple of the following brain-building practices to give yourself a better chance of avoiding cognitive decline.

Action Steps

Take on new projects to develop yourself. Join a book or discussion club or volunteer in your community. Read to kids at the library or visit the elderly in nursing or care homes. These activities also fulfill the need for quality social interaction.

Change your environment. Try new types of food or visit different communities. If you're financially able, travel. There is truly no better way to expand your brain and your mind.

Learn something that you've never thought about learning before. For example, learn a new language. Spanish and Mandarin are completely different, but they are the second and third most popular languages on the planet. How about studying one of them and planning a trip to where you can use that language? There are many incredible online courses these days on topics from mathematics to ancient civilizations, and many of them are very inexpensive. The Great Courses, Centre of Excellence, Udemy – all these platforms have many courses on many topics. You could spend the rest of your life learning new things right at home.

While online courses are great, there are also many community colleges and universities where you can audit courses for little or no money, especially if you're over 60. That way you will also meet new, most likely younger people who will give you a different outlook on life, and you will be stimulated by a new environment.

Learn to play a musical instrument. This is beneficial on many levels. Listening to music alone helps expand your brain, but by learning to play an instrument you are using your brain in an entirely different way. The complexities of hand movement combined with note-reading and timing engage many different parts of the brain, making them cooperate in ways they might never have before. I address this further in chapter 18.

So far there is little evidence that playing computerized brain games can improve broad cognitive abilities or increase the volume of the brain. But if you have never used a computer or played any kind of video game in the past, the act of learning how to do that can help with neuroplasticity.

Any new experience that requires mental effort produces changes in the neural systems used to acquire that new skill.[3] There could be an increase in the number of synapses or the number of neurons, or the connections between them could be strengthened. However, you can't keep playing the same video game, for example, and expect neuroplasticity to continue. You must keep learning.

Cognitive Reserve Can Be Developed Later in Life

As I mentioned in chapter 10, you develop cognitive reserve thanks to higher education, ongoing intellectual challenges, exposure to other cultures – that sort of thing. But just because you don't have a higher "formal" education, or you had a job that did not tax your brain, does not mean that you cannot nurture cognitive reserve later in life. Quite the opposite, in fact. The same things that nurture neuroplasticity also nurture cognitive reserve.

Spending quality active time with others is incredibly powerful. Studies have shown that seniors who engage in activities have a 38 percent reduction in the chance of suffering from dementia. If you can spend that active time in nature the effects are even greater, because being exposed to different plants and animals and being challenged by walking or climbing also help nurture cognitive reserve.

There are so many ways to grow and nurture your brain that there's no excuse to be bored. Turn off the TV and learn something new.

Chapter 17

Listening to the Sounds...
and the Silence

To understand how important sound and music are to your brain, let's start by understanding the importance of silence. Silence is much more than golden... it is regenerative.

Research into sounds and silence has found that prolonged silence can spur new cell development in the brain. Why exactly this occurs is not fully understood, but it could be because silence is such a rare commodity and is perceived as something new for the brain.

The most interesting study focused on mice, and while it wasn't conducted on humans, the results are very impressive. The researcher subjected three groups of adult mice to three types of sound: music, white noise, and infant mouse calls. A fourth group, which was supposed to be the control group, listened to two hours of silence per day. The first three groups experienced some positive effects, but nothing impressive or long-lasting. Amazingly, it was the control group that showed development of *new* brain cells in the hippocampus, which is the brain region that encodes new memories. The researcher hypothesized that the unusual experience of a silent environment prompted the mouse brains to increase in activity.[1]

Another study started out as an investigation into the efficacy of different kinds of music on reducing stress in people. A group of Italian researchers played short tracks of music in six different styles to human subjects. Between the tracks were segments of two minutes of silence. The researchers did not plan to investigate the effects of the pauses, but it turned out that the periods of two-minute silence produced a deeper state of relaxation in the participants than any kind of music.

One exciting learning tool has emerged from this research: When you are learning a new language (which is one of the best ways to help spur neuroplasticity), break your study time into 30-minute chunks. For the first few moments just sit in silence, relaxing, getting ready to learn. Spend the next 20 minutes or so studying. Then for the last five minutes, sit again in silence so that your learning has a chance to sink in.

Nurturing silence also helps you prepare for periods of meditation, which is covered in depth in chapter 20. It opens up space in your mind and heart to be more creative, including writing or music or art. Artistic expression is an incredibly powerful path to a healthy brain, so do nurture that silence.

Action Steps

If you can't stand the idea of being in your home without some kind of noise in the background, start your exploration into silence by doing simple things like making dinner and having your coffee without any music or television on in the background. Try walking or exercising without music or podcasts. For some of us that seems impossible, but you may find that it's a powerful way to notice and nurture the mind/body connection. Spend time in art galleries, libraries, or churches where stillness is the norm. It's a wonderful way to get used to quiet.

Over time you will begin to crave silence and nurture periods every day when silence reigns supreme. It helps you collect your thoughts, plan, dream, and simply enjoy being.

While silence is often golden, of course we also need auditory stimulation, and that's where music comes in with its powerful medicine.

Music for Your Mind

Music is much more than a diversion or a pleasant accompaniment to our lives. By listening mindfully, you can use music to enhance your ability to learn and to improve your health now, while protecting your brain for the future.

For Focus:

Think of the many things you learned as a child that were made easier with the use of rhyme and rhythm. For most of us the "Alphabet Song" made learning our ABCs much easier. That's because its simple rhythm and melody helped us stay focused as we mastered this fundamental task.

For Memory:

In contrast, if you want to improve memory, the best benefits come from listening to more complicated music such as classical music. In one interesting study Bulgarian psychologist George Lozanov found that background Baroque instrumental music by George Frideric Handel and Johann Sebastian Bach greatly increased learning and memory retention while learning a foreign language.

It seems this works because simultaneous activation of the left and right brain maximizes learning and retention of information. The information (the new language) being studied activates the left brain, while the music activates the right brain.

What music helps most? Anything with a 60-beat-per-minute pattern activates both sides of the brain in unison.[2] When I listen to such music I have to keep the volume low because, as a musician, I start analyzing the music. But this trick really helped me when I was studying for my nutritionist course.

For Neuroplasticity:

Another benefit of mindfully listening to music is encouraging neuroplasticity. One excellent brain-stimulating exercise is to choose an upbeat classical piece like the "Allegro" from Bach's Brandenburg Concerto No. 4 in G major.[3] While you're listening to the music, try to follow one part or one instrument. By doing this you're activating both halves of your brain in a way normally done only by musicians as they play their instrument.

For Emotional Support:

For calming and help with emotional problems, any music that evokes positive emotions helps increase blood flow to the brain. It has the same effect on the brain as the smell of lavender or chamomile, producing "feel-good" chemicals like dopamine. A 2011 study found that music plays a significant role in causing a good mood. It showed that dopamine levels were 9 percent higher in participants who listened to music they enjoyed.[4]

While listening to recorded music has many benefits, attending live concerts can be even more beneficial for the brain.[5] This is partly due to the power of connecting with others in a musical experience, and partly due to the live "presence" of the music.

For Treating Trauma and Post-Traumatic Stress Disorder (PTSD):

Trauma can create massive problems in your brain throughout your life, and if it remains unaddressed can be a major contributor to the development of dementia. PTSD, sexual or emotional abuse, growing up in a war zone – all of these and many more events, whether they occur in childhood or later in life, must be addressed to limit their effects on your brain. One of the best ways to do this is with music therapy, a clinically proven intervention that has been studied in over 3,000 research papers. It works.

If you have suffered trauma in any form, I highly recommend that you get treatment. While "talk" therapy can certainly help, many studies show that music therapy can be even more powerful than talking.[6]

Dealing with trauma in a healthy way, through meditation, mindfulness, and music therapy, can protect your brain from depression, anxiety, and all the other psychological and physical havoc wreaked by lingering and unresolved stress, which often contributes to the development of dementia. Please find a qualified therapist if you are dealing with these sorts of issues.

The Music of Memories

There is a fair amount of research showing that dementia patients, even those in advanced stages, respond positively to music that was popular when they were young, or that triggers memories for them. But you don't have to suffer from this disease to extract great benefit from listening to music that inspires memories. We are emotional beings – we need connections, and one way to bring people together is by listening to music together and sharing memories about what that music meant to us.

Spending time every week just sitting and listening to music you enjoy – perhaps music of your youth or something from a particularly happy experience – is a wonderful way to remember connections, even if it's a song that you enjoyed with someone you have lost.

The benefits are enhanced if you can talk with someone about it and reminisce together. (There's that powerful social interaction again!) Obviously you don't want to play music that exacerbates stress or depression, but exercising a memory through mindful listening can be hugely beneficial to your emotional health and, by extension, to your brain health.

Your Gut on Music

There is copious research about the effects of music on digestion and our ability to taste food and drink.[7]

Fast and loud music stimulates release of the stress hormone cortisol, which increases respiration and heart rate, taking energy away from proper digestion. And listening to this kind of music while eating distracts you from the flavors and textures of food, so you just gobble it down and don't even realize you're full.

Slower, quieter music promotes relaxation and slower eating, which means you chew your food more thoroughly and digest it more effectively. This leads to a happier, healthier microbiome. Eating more slowly also gives your stomach time to realize it's getting nourishment, so you feel full and stop eating – especially important if you are trying to lose weight to save your brain.

Action Steps

Be mindful of the music and other noise in your environment when you are eating. Mild classical or jazz at a background level is best for digestion.

Experiment with periods of silence when you are learning new things, whether it is studying an online course or learning a language.

Spend time just listening to music you enjoy. Try not to do anything else but mindfully pay attention to what's happening in the music, and notice if it inspires memories.

Chapter 18

The Creative Brain

We are spiritual beings with an innate need to create. Making music, painting, sculpting, writing, quilting, knitting… these are all pursuits that feed our souls. But they are much more than that. Creative endeavors of all kinds expand our minds and make our brains healthier and stronger. Let's start with my favorite.

Make Music

Dozens of studies have shown that no other art form, hobby, or activity can produce the same level of lasting neurological benefits as music. And these benefits are never out of reach. It doesn't matter when you start.

Play an Instrument

One powerful study followed twin pairs in which only one twin had dementia. The researchers controlled for sex, education, and physical activity, so the only difference was whether one twin played a musical instrument. Those who played were 36 percent less likely to develop dementia than the twin who did not play![1]

Problem-solving, memory, emotional intelligence, planning, and many more cognitive functions are enhanced by playing a musical instrument.[2] Learning to play an instrument also helps facilitate neuroplasticity,[3] and it is never too late to take up a musical instrument to help make structural and functional changes in your brain.

You're probably aware that your left brain is all about logic, math, objectivity, and reason while your right brain is more about the creative self. Because music is math, musicians use both sides of their brains all the time. And even when they are just listening to music, their brains work more symmetrically.[4]

The parts of musicians' brains responsible for motor control, auditory processing, and spatial coordination are larger and different from those of others. Even the corpus callosum, the broad band of nerve fibers that enables the two hemispheres of the brain to communicate with each other, is larger in musicians. This additional white matter may be why people who play music have more cognitive reserve, meaning that their brains are better able to withstand the ravages of time and the environment.

Musical training also improves everyday processing speed *and* working memory.[5] While many studies have shown that people reap the greatest benefits if they started playing at an early age, the great news is that it doesn't matter what instrument you choose or when you start to play.[6] The fact that you're learning and playing is hugely protective against dementia.

Drum

Drumming is almost magical for humans. That might be partly because it is in our genetic code. For millennia, humans have been drumming in ritual and for healing, to signal each other to gather, and to inspire fear or feelings of power in times of war. We respond to it in a primal fashion, but it is much more than emotional and cultural.[7] Our physical bodies, and particularly our brains, respond to drumming in incredible healing ways; and for dementia, Parkinson's, and stroke patients drumming can be a life-changer.

An interesting study was done with patients suffering from an inherited form of dementia, Huntington's disease (HD). In an effort to intervene early and delay clinical onset of the disease, researchers designed a pilot study using drumming and rhythm exercises. After two months of training there were improvements in executive function and changes in white-matter microstructure in participants' brains.[8] Drumming is not a cure, but this is one glimpse into the powerful effects of drumming even on a disease that is as relentless and resistant as HD.

Drumming helps protect our brains by demanding a degree of concentration. The drummer fixes their attention on one point of focus, the drum. This not only increases concentration, it also eliminates the "noise" and other stressors in their lives. Their minds can stay focused on the present, which is incredibly valuable in maintaining healthy brain function. The effect is magnified in a drumming circle, in which many people are focusing with intent on one thing, and the results are astounding.

There is a very cool website and blog by a drummer who offers some excellent tips for using the drum to reduce stress and improve your health.[9] I highly recommend that anyone who would like to get into drumming check it out.

Action Steps

If you played an instrument but haven't picked it up in years – have another go! Or choose one that appeals to you now. Lots of people are picking up ukuleles because they are fun, inexpensive, light, easy to take with you, and relatively simple to play. Folk harps are also great choices, although they're a bit more expensive. They're very intuitive to play, and if you played piano earlier in life it's an easy transition.

If you've never played an instrument – well, the world is your oyster! Choose something you've always dreamed of playing and... do it! If you can take lessons, even better. But if it's hard to find a teacher in your area, or budget is a problem, even a recorder or simple keyboard will do. It's all about using your brain in a *new* way. There are also countless online music schools now, and lots of free lessons as well.

Another great thing about musical training: The benefits accrue even if you already have early symptoms of cognitive decline. Studies have shown that the simple act of learning or playing an instrument can slow down and reverse some of the symptoms.

Sing

When you sing it activates a range of networks associated with memory, language, movement, listening, and planning.[10] Singing also triggers the release of dopamine and serotonin along with oxytocin, which alleviates anxiety and stress.

The benefits of singing regularly are cumulative, and it turns out that people who do so have reduced levels of cortisol, indicating lower stress. You do not have to have what society calls a "great voice" – just sing!

Singing with Others

Singing solo is great, but when you sing with others you get double the benefit. According to a new study on the benefits of singing among people with mental health conditions including anxiety and depression, researchers in the U.K. concluded that singing in groups could make you happier.[11] Since being happier leads to better mental health, and better mental health is an important component of preventing dementia, we can extrapolate that singing might help prevent dementia.

Singing in groups triggers actual physical changes that improve health by reducing cortisol and boosting the immune system.[12] Dozens of studies have demonstrated the improved quality of life and connection that singing even the most basic songs with others can offer.

Group singing is also a powerful way to connect with others by sharing emotions and memories. When singing together, the heartbeats of the singers synchronize.[13] That can be a powerful antidote to the loneliness and isolation often experienced by those who have retired and are left without many interests, or those who are already struggling with early dementia.

Action Steps

Sing like nobody's listening. Sing in the shower, in your car, on your walk – anywhere and anything. It's not about being a singer; it's about singing.

There is a powerful singing exercise that the editors of the Alzheimer's Prevention website claim can improve cognition and activate parts of the brain that are central to memory. It is called the Kirtan Kriya. Doing this practice for 12 minutes a day can improve cognition and activate parts of the brain that are central to memory.[14]

If you would like to sing in a group, there are many opportunities including church choirs, groups that go to nursing or care homes, and other community organizations.

Move to the Music

There are so many ways that dancing is good for your brain, it's tempting to just say, "Just go dancing," and leave you to figure it out. But I'll try to summarize.

To start with, it is an amazing way to get exercise. It combines aerobic fitness, sensorimotor skills, and cognitive demands while also having a low risk of incurring injuries.[15]

In one study that compared the benefits of dancing to those of traditional exercise, MRI brain scans showed that brain structure in the hippocampus was dramatically improved after participants participated in weekly choreographed dance routines. The study revealed that choreographed dance routines also boosted flexibility, endurance, and balance, all important in maintaining health as you age.[16]

In another 21-year-long study dances like the rumba and foxtrot that required two people to be in sync resulted in participants having a 76 percent reduction in the chance of getting Alzheimer's.[17] That result doesn't translate to free-form dancing, though. It's important to engage your brain while dancing. The act of concentrating while practicing the moves builds neuroplasticity, reminiscent of the benefits of learning a musical instrument.

Another way to benefit from dancing is through dance therapy, which has been proven to help people deal with trauma and reduce stress.

Action Steps

Dance to any kind of music that gets you to move your feet. If you can't move your feet, move your arms and your torso. Dance like nobody's watching; and even if somebody is, it doesn't matter.

For exercise-type dancing, there are many great videos on YouTube like those from Never Stop Dancing.[18]

Better yet, join a dance class at your local community center or gym, or take lessons. There are thankfully still places like Fred Astaire Dance Studios and countless others where you can learn with others. That way you're getting the benefit of the all-important social interaction along with the dancing.

To support you in using music to help save your memories, I've created Three Musical Hacks to Boost Your Brain. You can claim this free guide from my website at KateKunkel.com/the-book. Have fun!

Painting, Drawing, and Other Artistic Pursuits

Getting in touch with your creative muse is an incredibly powerful way to keep your brain healthy while boosting your emotional and spiritual health. The simple act of applying paint to canvas or doing a pencil sketch has been shown to relieve stress.

A study published by the *Journal of the American Art Therapy Association* compared saliva samples of 39 healthy individuals taken before and after 45 minutes of making art. Results showed that just engaging in the art-making activity significantly lowered cortisol levels and that the participants felt much more relaxed after the art session.[19]

Another benefit for older people comes in the form of improved cognitive and tactile abilities and subjective well-being from art-related activities. Art activities that enable people to work together are great ways to engage in social interaction, and they are believed to boost self-esteem and psychological health.

If you are already having some memory issues, creating art with colors can help. Painting boosts your memory skills, and people who are involved in drawing, writing, and painting are at lower risk of developing memory-related illnesses during their older age.

All that aside, creative expression is a great way to exercise your mind, express emotions, and nurture your spiritual self, all of which are essential for brain health.

Writing can also be incredibly therapeutic. Many people write poetry as a way to express emotions that cannot otherwise be shared, and journaling is an excellent way to handle stress. By mixing images and words, sketching, painting, coloring, and writing poems, people are creating beautiful books that help strengthen their memories now and act as reminders of a life well lived.

Action Steps

While it seems rudimentary, simply coloring mandalas or images in adult coloring books is a great brain-booster. Choosing colors and seeing how the images come together is excellent stress reduction. The same goes for the great new paint-by-number kits now available.

There are countless art classes online and in local communities – take one! Just play with the colors and the different media and have fun. It's not about being an "artist" – it's about expressing yourself.

Start journaling. I recommend journaling your way through the Eight Weeks to a Better Brain program. It will help you keep track of how you are feeling, and it might just spur you to write more. You probably have a powerful story in there somewhere; perhaps this will help you find your voice.

Expressing yourself through music, dance, art, and even crafts touches so many of the points that help protect our brains that I cannot stress it enough. Don't let "perfection paralysis" stop you. Just enjoy!

Chapter 19

Alternative and Complementary Therapies

When we are being proactive and working to prevent any disease, whether it is cancer or Alzheimer's, a multifaceted approach always works best.

So far, we've covered the essentials: a whole-foods, plant-based diet; reducing toxins; getting more exercise and better sleep; reducing stress; and keeping our brains challenged. But there are many other, what might be considered alternative, therapies that can offer substantial benefits.

These are not included in the Eight Weeks to a Better Brain program itself because it can be difficult to get access to light or vibroacoustic or similar therapies where you are, but there is good research indicating they can help protect your brain. If you find something of interest and you get an opportunity to try it, go for it!

Aromatherapy

For many people the idea of using essential oils for treatment of dementia fits right in there with bloodletting and leeches. But there is copious research confirming the benefits of essential oils for memory and cognition.[1] They are also powerful for those who have no signs of cognitive decline but suffer from stress, depression, or cardiovascular issues, all of which can contribute to the likelihood of developing dementia. We'll cover just a few of the most well-researched aromatherapy oils.

Rosemary

Rosemary as an herb is powerful for cognition, and you can read more about that in chapter 12. Using it in aromatherapy is also proving to be effective. In one study researchers exposed subjects to the aroma of rosemary while they were doing mathematical and visual-processing tasks. The stronger the rosemary aroma, the faster and more accurately the subjects performed their tasks! Mood also improved.[2] In another study researchers found that school-aged children who were placed in a room infused with rosemary had significantly higher memory scores than children who were in a room without the scent.[3]

There is no clear reason why it works. Some speculate that it stimulates electrical activity in the brain or that the pharmacologically active compounds can be absorbed and cause chemical reactions. To me all that matters is it works, and it can't hurt!

In another study researchers gave rosemary water to subjects given tasks to perform.[4] Ingestion of the water enhanced memory-based aspects of cognitive function, improved alertness, and reduced stress. There was also an indication that it delivered cardiovascular benefits.

In addition to using rosemary in foods and making a tea from it, you can infuse rosemary oil in the room where you are working or studying.

Lavender

Lavender essential oil has long been used to alleviate stress, headaches,[5] depression, and anxiety, all of which fall under the umbrella of neurological conditions.[6]

In 2010 the *International Journal of Psychiatry in Clinical Practice* confirmed lavender oil's efficacy in seven separate trials.[7] In one case, lavender oil ingested in a capsule was shown to consistently relieve symptoms such as sleep disturbance and anxiety and improve the quality of life for those with these conditions.[8] Even better, no one reported side effects, interactions, or withdrawal symptoms, unlike with pharmaceuticals that are used for the same conditions.

A 2012 study from Germany demonstrated the restorative benefits of inhaled lavender essential oil vapor. Patients with dementia inhaled lavender for 60 minutes a day, resulting in significantly improved sleep, moods, and health. Individuals with PTSD reported reduced states of depression.[9]

Lavender can be used in a multitude of ways including topically (with a carrier oil) and by diffusing, and lavender buds can be eaten.

Frankincense

In a 2013 meta-study, the authors cited several studies that showed that frankincense can help improve memory. The study authors believe frankincense aids in increasing the number of dendritic segments and branching in the neurons of the hippocampus, creating more synaptic connections, which therefore improve learning and memory.[10] It has also been shown to improve mood and have a calming effect, all important for a happy brain.

For calming and improving mood, one or two drops of frankincense essential oil directly on the skin at the wrist works well. Frankincense oil can also be ingested – three or four drops in a capsule or in a teaspoon of maple syrup.

There are certainly other essential oils, like the citrus-based essential oils and bergamot, that are helpful in reducing stress. One study found that bergamot aromatherapy helped increase the level of GABA in the right hippocampus, helping to ease anxiety.[11] Other studies found that bergamot increased focus, which can help with anxiety and stress.

Research is ongoing for using essential oils for gut health, and since our brains and guts are so intimately related, I believe this is an area that deserves more attention. Clove, ginger, cardamom, caraway, thyme, oregano, and peppermint oils have all been used to help alleviate symptoms of leaky gut.[12] Fennel and cumin are also used to alleviate irritable bowel syndrome (IBS) and help prevent symptoms of poor digestion.[13]

It would take an entire book to cover all the ways aromatherapy could help prevent dementia, so if using them appeals to you, I recommend talking to a qualified aromatherapist.

Heat, Cold, and Saunas

Heat Therapy

In chapter 14 you learned about autophagy, which is the cleaning-up of old and damaged cells. It happens throughout the body, but in the brain it is especially important. Besides fasting, another powerful way to support brain autophagy is through heat therapy. The stress of the heat urges your body to destroy old and damaged cells and create new and healthy cells. One way to achieve heat therapy is by using a sauna.

Sitting in a sauna makes you sweat, which itself is powerful for detoxification. But beyond that, the heat also helps open blood vessels, which allows more blood to flow to your brain so it can nourish, detoxify, and clean out the old or damaged cells.

Using a sauna can help promote weight loss and reverse the cardiovascular disease that leads to strokes and heart attacks. Fifteen minutes in an infrared sauna each day for 14 days has been shown to boost artery function by 40 percent, and enjoying a sauna also helps reduce inflammation.

But it's not just heat that can do all this fantastic work. While the Scandinavian tradition of taking hot saunas and then plunging into cold water seems bizarre to many of us, research has shown that this hot and cold therapy is beneficial to the brain. This is partly because it helps stimulate the production of brain-derived neurotrophic factor (BDNF), which is involved in neuron and brain-cell growth.

Cold Therapy

Cold therapy also helps increase brain autophagy.[14] As with heat therapy, the stress from the cold leads to autophagy and the creation of new and healthy cells.

It is believed that cold therapy may also increase mental focus due to the release of catecholamine it provides. Exposure to cold activates the sympathetic nervous system and increases endorphins (our feel-good neurotransmitters). It also increases the release of noradrenaline in the brain, which prepares the body for action and sharpens focus.

Because we have many cold receptors in our skin, exposure to cold sends electrical impulses to the brain, which some studies suggest result in an anti-depressant effect.

Cold therapy methods include cryotherapy chambers, jumping into a cold pool, and taking a cold shower.

Research indicates that the best results for the brain come from combining hot and cold therapy. A simple way to achieve this is by finishing up your very warm shower with a cold shower, and be sure to get your head wet with the cold water.

Light Therapy

There are five different types of bioactive light that help protect your brain.

- Far infrared, which is what is used in most red-light saunas, acts to heat up your cells. It mimics the part of the sun's spectrum that you feel as heat. It stimulates changes in cell function and circulation.
- Red light stimulates increased cellular energy through the production of adenosine triphosphate (ATP) by acting on the mitochondria in your cells.
- Near-infrared light works in basically the same way as red light to stimulate ATP production.
- Blue light is responsible for setting the circadian rhythm in your brain, and thereby regulates various hormones and transmitters. This is one reason so many people have trouble sleeping these days; there is too much artificial blue light from our electronic devices.
- UV light allows you to synthesize vitamin D_3 from the sun, and you have already learned that vitamin D deficiency is a huge contributor to cognitive decline.

Studies have shown improvements in cognitive performance and memory,[15] improved brain function after traumatic brain injury, improved mood, and improvements in mitochondrial function through use of red light. Red light also addresses hypoperfusion, which is when body tissues don't receive enough oxygen and nutrients. If this is left unchecked, tissues, including brain tissue, will die.

As you now know, inflammation is a huge contributor to the likelihood of developing dementia. This is partly because, when a neuron fires, there is an increase of about 40 percent in blood flow; however, only 4 percent of that 40 percent is needed to recharge the neuron. The rest of the blood flow works to reduce and remove heat from the neuron; it acts kind of like the coolant in a radiator. But if there is too much inflammation, the neurons cannot be cooled down and damage occurs, leading eventually to brain dysfunction.

There is, however, a way to use red and near-infrared light to stimulate healing, relieve pain and inflammation, and prevent tissue from dying. It's called photobiomodulation. The following explanation of photobiomodulation is rudimentary, but I hope you get the idea. If you'd like to read a more scientific explanation, the paper referenced has a detailed explanation.[16]

In one product from Canada, the patient wears a helmet-like structure with clusters of light-emitting arrays set at 40 hertz (Hz). The light from these clusters targets specific sections of the brain known to work together. The therapy energizes the mitochondria, the energy centers of the cells. In this system there is also a nasal lens emitting at 10 Hz that targets the underside of the brain.[17]

This light therapy has resulted in changes in the functional, behavioral, emotional, and cognitive behaviors of people after one six-minute treatment, and intensive treatment has shown significant reversals in their symptoms. However, the benefits lasted only if they continued to receive the treatment.

For prevention, infrared light could help stave off or delay symptoms of dementia.

I believe the best way to use light therapeutically is by getting outside in the sun, but if you have some memory or focus issues, intense therapy like this could be an option.

Vibroacoustic Therapy

It might be hard to understand how pure sound can help prevent dementia, but the amazing fact is – it can.

Vibroacoustic therapy (VAT)[18] uses specific sound frequencies (not music) to produce vibrations that are applied directly to the body. During the vibroacoustic therapy process, a client lies on a specially designed mat or bed or sits in a chair that is embedded with speakers or transducers that transmit sound into vibrations that travel through the body.

VAT has been used to successfully treat many conditions including chronic pain and fibromyalgia, and it is awesome for stress reduction. It is also used to treat people who have Parkinson's to significantly reduce anxiety and tremors, and people who have Alzheimer's to help them connect with the present.

Studies from the 1990s showed that an internal brain rhythm of 40 Hz is a fundamental frequency in a healthy brain. This frequency is called *gamma*. Gamma waves are the fastest brain activity[19] and are responsible for cognitive function, learning, memory, and information processing.[20]

Recent studies have shown great promise in stimulating gamma-wave activity in the brain[21] with vibroacoustic therapy. In a study by Dr. Lee Bartel of Toronto, 18 patients with mild to severe Alzheimer's disease sat for 30-minute sessions, twice per week, in a vibroacoustic chair with a 40 Hz frequency program being delivered through the chair.

At the end of the three-week study patients scored on average nearly four points higher on a 30-point cognitive function scale. As is the case with most treatments for Alzheimer's patients, those with late-stage Alzheimer's showed minimal improvement. Mild to mid-stage patients had more improvement, but the benefits faded within a week of the last session.[22]

To me this means that this therapy holds great potential, but you must start early and keep using the therapy. If you combine this therapy with better nutrition, exercise, and social interaction, the benefits will be much greater, and if you do it before there are cognitive issues it will help prevent the slide into dementia.

The wonderful thing about VAT is that you can buy a cushion[23] or a lounge[24] to use at home.

I have been using and administering vibroacoustic therapy since 2001, and I believe it is one of the best kept secrets in alternative therapies. That it helps patients with cognitive issues is the icing on the cake for me.

Even if you are not exhibiting signs of cognitive decline now, it's one of the many tools you can use right away to get into the peaceful, relaxed state that is so important for brain health.

CBD Oil

In ongoing research, cannabidiol (CBD oil) has been shown to reduce or remove the impacts of inflammation, oxygen buildup, and brain cell decline.[25]

Inflammation increases when the brain's immune cells are unable to clear disorienting blockages, but this effect can be reduced by using CBD oil. It is also an antioxidant, so it helps reduce the problems associated with oxygen stress.

In a 2011 study by Australian researchers, CBD oil was also shown to stimulate the growth and development of brain cells, consequently reducing the decline of memory and other brain functions.[26]

As this product has been approved for use in many countries now, it may be something to consider in order to help nurture the growth of brain cells.

Hyperbaric Oxygen Therapy

Hyperbaric oxygen therapy has been shown to support brain autophagy. It also helps raise the level of oxygen in tissues, supports new blood vessel growth, and increases production of stem cells.

To learn more about hyperbaric oxygen therapy, I recommend reading "The Health Benefits of HyperBaric Oxygen Therapy" by Dr. David Jockers and following the research he cites.[27]

&

These are just a few of the many complementary therapies you can use to enhance the steps in the Eight Weeks to a Better Brain program. They may be especially helpful if you are already dealing with memory, focus, or personality-change issues. If any of them appeal to you I encourage you to do your own further research.

> *If you want to stay on top of emerging therapies, be sure to check out my blog at **KateKunkel.com**. I keep a close eye on new developments and continually share them with my readers.*

Chapter 20

Mindfulness, Meditation, and Spirituality

While you can do a great deal to protect your brain by eating healthily, exercising, and getting quality sleep, you are not just a physical being; you are a spiritual being. And this side of you must also be nurtured for your brain to be healthy and your mind to be whole.

In chapter 8 I listed a few meditation practices that can help, and I expand on them here. But let's start with mindfulness, something that is incredibly easy, although you might find it challenging at first.

Mindfulness

One of the most powerful practices to nurture your heart is mindfulness, which is the nonjudgmental awareness of experiences in the present moment. Many studies have shown that mindfulness creates numerous health benefits, and while the exact mechanism is not totally understood,[1] we do know that in addition to helping reduce stress (a huge contributor to dementia risk), it increases grey matter.[2]

There are four basic ways that mindfulness helps your brain:

1. **By regulating attention:** If you train your brain to come back to the present, you can maintain awareness about whatever you're doing and observe any emotions that arise while you are engaged. This practice can help you develop more positive emotions – something essential for brain health.

2. **By bringing awareness to your body's sensations:** This helps you maintain your mind/body connection and foster emotional awareness and regulation.

3. **By helping you alter your self-perceptions:** Mindfulness helps you see that you are continually changing, which helps you lose your attachment to outcomes and to your entrenched patterns of behavior. If you can lose those attachments you tend to be happier. Happier person – healthier brain.

4. **By helping you regulate your emotional responses:** Mindfulness helps you accept that it's okay to have bodily responses to emotional experiences while also realizing that you don't have to react to those responses. It helps you release judgment and facilitates a feeling of well-being.

So how do you achieve this mindfulness? Well, to start with, it's important to understand that mindfulness is not a destination. It's a journey. By incorporating mindful attention in your daily life, whether it's doing the dishes, sitting in traffic, or sitting on your meditation cushion, you become more settled and content.

These seven elements of mindfulness are attributed to Jon Kabat-Zinn, but I adapted them specifically to address the health of your brain:

1. **Beginner's Mind**

    Cultivating a beginner's mind means you are willing to view everything as if for the very first time – the joy, the feeling, the uniqueness of every moment and every experience.

    Every time you do something, even if you've done it a thousand times, can you do it with a fresh view? Is there something new to be noticed? Don't let what you think you know prevent you from seeing things as they truly are.

2. **Non-Judging**

    To practice non-judging, try going through a day paying attention to how often you judge things that come into your experience, whether it's someone who is taking too long to pay at the grocery store or how you react to something on social media.

Consider what it would be like to simply experience and observe these events without clinging to judging whether they are good or bad. See what it feels like to be an impartial witness to the experience. The goal is not necessarily to try to stop judging (though that is a worthy effort), but just to be *aware* that you're doing it.

3. **Patience**

What does *patience* really mean? Do you practice patience with a feeling of long-suffering and endurance, or can you practice it with a feeling of deep faith in yourself and in life?

Let everything unfold in its time; don't be in such a hurry to get through one thing to move on to the next one.

4. **Trust**

It is important to trust yourself. Many of us have given our power away to an outside authority: a teacher, a boss, or the government. But by meditating and becoming mindful you can access your own wisdom, knowledge, and skill.

Strive to pay attention to thoughts of self-doubt when they arise and look deeply into where they really come from instead of just believing them. Trust yourself.

5. **Non-Striving**

This is probably one of the most difficult elements of mindfulness to grasp and incorporate into your life. A good example is when you begin to meditate. You might think or say, "I don't think I meditate correctly," but there really is no "correct" way to meditate. If you are only focusing on doing it right, then you will always be questioning yourself and not actually enjoying what you are doing or experiencing. It's the same with anything you might be learning or doing.

Try simply *being with* what you're doing rather than striving to do it.

6. **Acceptance**

Practicing non-striving leads you directly to the next attitudinal quality of mindfulness, which is acceptance. Sometimes we confuse acceptance with approval or resignation. But *accepting* just means seeing something as it is right now; it doesn't mean you aren't going to do something about it if it isn't in your best interests.

Accept where you are, how you are. No one ever changed by hating themselves into it. And that includes creating a lifestyle that is good for your brain.

7. **Letting Go**

This last quality is built on and includes all the elements discussed above. Hopefully you have experienced moments of letting go in your life – perhaps when spending time with a child, or, if you are a musician, getting completely lost in your music.

For many of us this doesn't happen often, but when it does – wow – it's just wonderful. That's letting go. As you become more mindful, you'll be able to set aside judgment of yourself and what happens to you in life, which means it will be easier to let things go. Then you have room for all the wonder of new things, including a lifestyle that saves your brain.

Meditation

There are literally dozens of forms of meditation, from focused attention on a light or sound to transcendental meditation to breathing meditation. The way you meditate is not as important as the fact that you meditate, and that you make it a part of your everyday life.

Focus Meditation

Focus meditation is also called concentration meditation. It teaches you to focus your mind and turn off that "monkey mind" that we all seem to deal with from time to time. You can focus on a sound like a gong or recorded music, a candle, a piece of art, or tactile sensations like mala beads. You can also focus on taste or smell, or even your breath.[3]

> *As you add meditation to your brain-healthy lifestyle, it often helps to have a contemplative piece of music upon which you can focus. I would like to offer you a gift to help with this. It is a 15-minute solo harp piece that I improvised in a meditation, for meditation. You can claim it at KateKunkel.com/the-book.*

Heart-Centered Meditation

In heart-centered meditation you quiet your mind and bring awareness to the energy center in the middle of your chest – your heart. You focus on your heart's influence on your true self, with the idea of unifying mind, body, and spirit.

Tai Chi[4] and Qigong[5]

These are immensely popular for people who just can't sit still. These are moving meditations that combine physical exercise with breathing and focus and sometimes sound.

Yoga[6]

While many people think of yoga as a physical exercise, and it is that too, yoga is more than just acquiring and holding a pose. It involves quieting your inner-most thoughts and being in the moment while forging a connection between your mind and body. Pranayama is a form of yoga that focuses on the formal practice of controlling the breath, which is the source of our *prana*, or vital life force. The somewhat formal practices in this kind of yoga are great if you have trouble just "sitting there."

Transcendental Meditation[7]

This is a technique to help you avoid distracting thoughts using a mantra – which is a word, phrase, or sound – to promote a state of relaxed awareness. For the formal training, you work with a trained teacher. But you can do similar forms of mantra-based meditation on your own.

Walking Meditation

A walking meditation has you breathing in time with your footsteps and turning your focus to the connection between your body and mind.

ॐ

It really doesn't matter how you meditate, what technique you use, or even how long you do it, especially at first. If you can sit still for or commit to only five minutes a day – that's better than nothing, right? And if you can't sit, try walking meditation or qigong. The thing is to be consistent. Try to do it at the same time and in the same place every day. Habit-forming is essential for success in meditation.

I like to meditate at night so that I am relaxed to get that all-important sleep. But many people prefer doing it in the morning to start the day in a calm state. You might have to experiment a bit, but you will find what works for you.

Spirituality, Your Heart, and Your Brain

Many people have difficulty imagining that spirituality has anything to do with brain health. But it is vital, and that's why I spend a lot of time talking about fostering your creative side by writing or doing art or music or anything else that gives you an opportunity to express yourself (chapter 18).

Beyond those expressions, though, a healthy spiritual life has been shown to help protect your brain and your mind in numerous ways. There is a field of study called *neurotheology* which studies the spiritual brain. One study found that the brains of Buddhist monks who have been practicing meditation for years undergo less neuronal aging than those of laypeople. Buddhist monks also develop greater resistance to the feeling of pain, and retain information and memories longer than the average person.

Spirituality is by its very nature different for everyone, but generally it has these components:

- Having a sense of purpose in life
- Being able to spend time to think and just "be"
- Taking time to reflect on life events and their meanings
- Understanding and articulating what you believe in

- Caring for others
- Practicing forgiveness and compassion
- Recognizing right and wrong and acting accordingly

Incorporating altruism, forgiveness, and a sense of purpose into your life has a positive impact on your physical and emotional health, and thus on your brain. Part of that can be explained simply by the stress reduction, but these attitudes have also been shown to have a positive impact on blood pressure and heart rate,[8] which are of course related to brain health.[9]

In the Baltimore Longitudinal Study on Aging,[10] results showed that the attitude people had toward aging itself made a significant difference in the brains of the participants, who were all dementia-free when the study began. People who initially had more negative views of aging had a significantly greater buildup of the amyloid plaques and neurofibrillary tangles that are the markers of Alzheimer's compared with those who had more positive attitudes. Another study showed that people with such negative views also had more shrinkage in the hippocampus.[11]

&

A positive outlook on life and aging and a contemplative practice of some kind, whether it's mindfulness or meditation or a religious tradition, are important practices that will help you improve your health (and your life) now, and save your brain for the future.

Closing Thoughts

I hope that what you've learned in *Don't Let the Memories Fade* has convinced you that you do have control over your health and your brain and that by incorporating the Eight Weeks to a Better Brain program into your lifestyle, you are creating a healthier and more vibrant future.

If you kept a journal while you were doing the program, do keep it up. That will help you keep track of your successes, frustrations, and what you like and don't like about the recipes and meals. As you try more new foods and experiment with natural cleaning products, exercises, and the like, you'll have a record of what did and did not work for you so you can refer back as you progress.

To get support as you continue your new lifestyle, please join our **Prevent Dementia with Music, Mind and Matter Facebook group.** It is a great community where you can learn more about diet and exercise, and where we share recipes and tips that we learn along the way. You will also get support when life events challenge your resolve to look after yourself.

You might "fall off the wagon" from time to time. Heaven knows I have! Sometimes I just have to have a beer and some corn chips, but the next day I get right back to my kombucha and carrots. (Well, no, not exactly, but you get what I mean.) This is the kind of thing that we share and support each other about on the Facebook group.

I do hope you'll join us there so we can play together in this wonderful adventure that will make sure you *don't let the memories fade.*

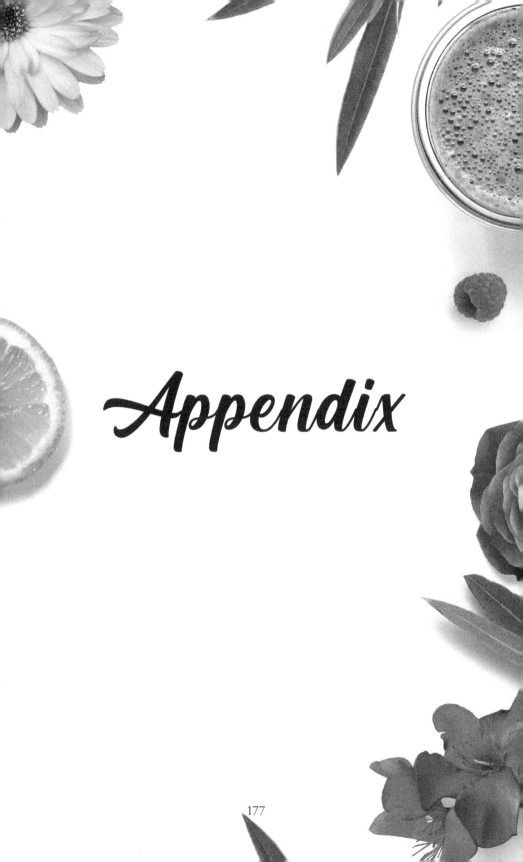

Appendix

Contents

Resources for Weeks One to Eight in the Program

In chapter 11 there are references to online resources designed to help you enhance the benefits of this program. This is where you will find them, along with additional references that could be of interest and value.

Week One:

This week we're eliminating sugar. This may be a bit more difficult than you might imagine because there are 61 different names for sugar! It can be hiding in many places. While you probably know the most common names, there are some that are confusing, like demerara sugar, dextrin, dextrose, glucose, glucose solids, HFCS (high-fructose corn syrup), maltodextrin, maltol, maltose, mannose, muscovado, panocha, refiner's syrup, rice syrup, saccharose, sorghum syrup, sucrose, sweet sorghum, and treacle.

There are good resources online to check if you're not quite sure, so refer to them to learn all the different names this sweet poison can hide under.

For musical meditation: To obtain a free recording of harp meditation music, go to *https://katekunkel.com/the-book*. There you will see a link to claim your music.

There are many good, free sources for gentle qigong exercises. One low source is on You Tube, on the channel *'Eight Pieces'*.

Week Two:

The Sauerkraut recipe is under Fermented Foods (#2).

Recipes for the Natural Cleaning Products are at the end of the appendix.

You can find many morning yoga routines online, but one 10-minute morning yoga I enjoy is also on You Tube, at '*Yoga by Candace*'. Lots of great free content there.

Week Three:

The Vegan "Alfredo" Sauce recipe is under Dinner Recipes (#3).

This week you begin to incorporate kombucha and/or kefir water. If you wish to make your own, starter kits can be purchased at *Cultures for Health* online. I have no affiliation, it's just where I buy mine.

For tai chi: There is an excellent introductory lesson on You Tube at '*Taiflow*'.

Week Four:

Starting Fermented Foods – you will have 4 to 8 ounces of kombucha and/or kefir water PLUS one forkful of sauerkraut or kimchi every day. The Simple Cabbage Kimchi recipe is under Fermented Foods in the appendix (#3).

Meditations: *Sounds True* has three free meditations on the platform's website, but there are countless good meditations online.

For learning new things: *Udemy, Centre of Excellence,* and *The Great Courses* are three great platforms offering reasonably priced online courses in many fields. You're sure to find something you like in one of them!

Week Five:

Dr. *⸱⸱⸱* ou will start time-restricted eating, or intermittent fasting. There *⸱⸱⸱*ion about this at the *Amen brain health* website, and also on

Purposeful Listening for Learning: There is one particular *Brandenburg Concerto - No. 6 in B Flat Major BWV 1051*. The music is complex enough to give your brain a workout. Try to follow the principal violin or choose another instrument. This makes your brain work like that of a musician and is excellent for neuroplasticity.

Week Six:

Learning Music: There are so many options, it can be a bit confusing if you haven't played much before. I went through several sites and found these that seem among the best.

If you're considering playing piano, there is a site called *Piano Nanny* that has good starter lessons.

There are many good sources of free harp lessons, including one resource at *Harp Fandom* where they have gone through the trouble of analyzing good lessons. I am a harp teacher, so if you have any questions, you can always reach out to me through my website at *KateKunkel.com*.

You can find lessons for just about every instrument you want to learn online, but I do encourage personal lessons if you can manage it. Remember that all-important social interaction!

Week Seven:

Art Therapy: *Udemy* and *The Great Courses* both have many art programs available.

Week Eight:

If you are interested in vibroacoustic (sound) therapy, visit *VibroacousticTherapy. com*. Lots of information there!

Introduction to the Meal Plans and Recipes

Instead of following rigid weekly meal plans, this program allows you to mix and match meals from lunches and dinners and breakfasts.

The only things that should be incorporated *every day* to give you the best results are:

Start every day with lemon, cider vinegar, or rosemary water.

From Week 3 you'll add kombucha or kefir water every day. (4 to 8 ounces each day)

From Week 4 you'll add a small serving of fermented vegetables (in the form of sauerkraut or kimchi) to one meal a day. Just a forkful each day is enough, especially at first.

Everything else is your choice, and I encourage you to mix it up.

The lunches here are items you can make the night or day before. That way, if you are taking lunch with you to an outside job, you will have a meal that is nutritious and travels well.

These recipes have been chosen for ingredients that help reduce inflammation, improve insulin sensitivity, and feed your brain. However, I did not create menus, so you may want to add salads or other side dishes to enhance some of your meals. Please just don't add white rice or bread, or processed salad dressings.

The Meal Plan Jumble is arranged simply by Breakfast, Lunch, and Dinner and you will find the numbered recipes in the appropriate pages in the Recipes section. In addition to those entrees, you will also find recipes for Soups and Stews, Snacks and Appetizers, International Flavors, and Desserts and Sweet Energy Treats.

Be sure to note the Vegan Basics because that is where you will find recipes for Vegan Butter, cheeses, and other essentials that you will use often.

Everything uses ingredients that are on your "Foods to Eat" list, and every recipe has been tested by me. Some are my own creations; some are adapted from other sources. The ones I've offered are a good place to start your whole-foods, plant-based, brain-healthy lifestyle.

Pantry List

These are the ingredients we use most often in this program.

You probably already have many of the spices and basics. You do not have to get everything at once; this list is the ultimate for a full-stocked pantry.

Spend some time looking over the recipes and see what appeals to you for the first week, then create your personalized shopping list based on those dishes.

Beverages

Coffee (organic and fair trade if possible)
Teas (black, green, matcha, herb, whatever you like)
Kombucha tea

Cereals/grains and grain replacements

Almond flour
Almond meal
Brown rice flour (be sure this is organic)
Coconut flour
Oats – not quick oats – gluten free and organic
Quinoa
Tapioca and/or cassava (yucca) flour
Wild rice

Dried/canned goods

Black beans – 2 cans or one large bag dried
Garbanzo beans (chickpeas) – 3 cans or one large bag dried
White beans – one can
Coconut milk, full fat – 3 cans
Cacao powder – 100% pure, no sugar
Lentils – red and green or brown
Pasta – chia, quinoa, or other gluten-free, grain-free
Vegetable broth (in Tetra Pak) – low sodium, organic (if you don't have the time to make your own broth)
Dried Fruits: Raisins
    Apricots
    Cranberries
    Dates

Optional: Preserved tomatoes (canned tomatoes are risky because of the liners, whether or not they have BPA, so I don't recommend them). Tetra Pak is a carton-type packaging currently used by Pomi. A better choice is your own preserved tomatoes, or those that come in glass jars, if you can find them. Most of the recipes use fresh tomatoes.

Oils

Avocado oil
Coconut oil –two kinds - organic, virgin AND refined (for some recipes)
Olive oil – organic, extra virgin, pure (check sources)

Refrigerated section

Almond and/or or hemp milk, unsweetened
Organic tempeh
Organic tofu
Plant-based yogurt – unsweetened, unflavored

Seeds/Nuts

Almonds
Cashews (raw)
Chia seeds
Flax seeds (Flax meal is also fine, but the seeds last longer. You can grind them into meal as you need it for recipes.)
Sesame seeds
Sunflower seeds (raw)
Walnuts

Spices (organic, if possible)

Black pepper
Cinnamon
Cloves
Coriander
Cumin
Curry powder
Garlic powder
Ginger powder
Onion powder
Rosemary
Thyme
Turmeric

Staples

Apple cider vinegar
Baking soda
Baking powder – aluminum free
Himalayan pink salt (also called Himalayan salt or just pink salt)
Maple syrup
Nutritional yeast (be sure it has vitamin B_{12} added)
Peppercorns
Psyllium husk
White vinegar

Vegetable bouillon cubes (organic)

Optional: Probiotic capsules (if you plan on making plant-based yogurt – or you can just buy one container of the yogurt from the store)

The Meal Plan Jumble

Every Day before Breakfast:

Have a cup of warm water with lemon or apple cider vinegar or a cup of rosemary water. It's best to make rosemary water the night before by pouring boiling water over a sprig of rosemary and letting it steep overnight. Strain out the herb and drink. You can also use dried rosemary.

Tea or coffee – clear or black or with plant-based milks.

Breakfast Choices

1. Smoothies – so many choices, just mix and match to what you have on hand and what you feel like every day
2. Banana Pancakes
3. Garbanzo Bean Scramble
4. Vegan Frittata (for days when you have a lot of time, or for Sunday brunch)
5. Buckwheat Apple Muesli
6. Ginger Spiced Tofu Pancakes
7. Sweet Potato Anti-Inflammatory Muffins – great to make ahead and freeze

Lunch Choices

1. NotEgg Salad wrap or sandwich
2. Bowl Lunches
3. Quinoa Tabbouleh

4. Green Beans and Cherry Tomato Salad
5. Potato and Sun-Dried Tomato Salad
6. Curried Tofu Salad
7. The Best Change-It-Up Broccoli Salad

Many of the offerings in Salads are great for lunch, and many can be made up to two days ahead of time, so be sure to explore those as well.

Dinner Choices

1. Broccoli Mushroom Curry and Beans
2. Brain-Boosting Black Beans, Quinoa, and Zucchini
3. Veggie "Pasta" with Vegan "Alfredo" Sauce (noted in Week 4 of the Program in chapter 11)
4. Sesame Tempeh Stir-Fry
5. Veggie and Tahini Bake
6. Tempeh Bolognese
7. Mushroom Cauliflower Risotto
8. Portobello Mushrooms Stuffed with Broccoli and Spinach
9. Lentil Shepherd's Pie

Note: Any of the Soups and Stews or the Salads also make great dinners. Just be sure you're getting enough calories per day. And if you're not 100 percent certain you're getting enough nutrients (review chapter 15), be sure to supplement.

Remember: Starting in Week 4 – add a forkful of sauerkraut or kimchi to your meals. Or just have some as a snack.

Recipes

Breakfasts and Brunches

1. Smoothies

Smoothies can be made with basically anything you like depending on what fruits, vegetables, seeds, and superfoods you have on hand. (I recommend NOT using purple or red cabbage. Lesson learned!)

Smoothies are also a great way to use up bananas and avocados that are getting close to overripe. Components of a smoothie that is particularly good for your brain:

i. A green leafy vegetable:

…like kale, spinach, chard, dandelion greens (For these, it's important that you seek out organic, because spinach and kale are among the most pesticide-laden veggies.)

ii. A superfruit:

…like berries or dark cherries. I classify avocado here as well, because it truly is a superfruit, AND it has healthy fats.

In North America it's relatively easy to find frozen blueberries and other fruits, so this is a good option off-season. And here again, beware of the dirty dozen. Strawberries are heavily sprayed, so try for organic. I put raw cacao in here, because it is a superfruit, even though we don't think of it as a fruit. If you're making a smoothie featuring plant-based milks, this is a natural.

iii. Something to add a touch of sweetness

...like bananas, pears, dates

iv. A source of liquid

Coconut water is my favorite but depending on whatever else you have for ingredients, you can use plant-based milks or even watermelon juice.

v. A source of protein

... like peanut, cashew, or almond butter: or pieces of nuts, seeds

Other tasty additions that are good for your brain: Ginger, cinnamon, vanilla

2. Banana Pancakes

Ingredients:

- 1 very ripe large banana (or two very small bananas)
- 1 cup almond milk
- 1 cup almond flour

Directions:

Mash the banana, add the milk and flour, and mix until there are no lumps. I use a high-speed blender, but you can certainly do it with a fork.

Put a few drops of coconut oil in a safe non-stick pan – warm until a flick of water makes the oil sputter.

Add 3 tablespoons of batter to the pan and fry – once the top starts to bubble, flip the pancake over and cook until golden brown. Repeat until the batter is used up.

Serve with fruit and/or whipped coconut cream.

Optional additions: chia seeds or ground flax seed for additional omega-3

3. Garbanzo Bean Scramble

Ingredients:

- 2 cups (330g) canned garbanzo beans, drained
- ½ tsp. turmeric
- ½ tsp. paprika
- 2 tsp. olive oil
- 1 small onion, finely diced
- 2 cloves garlic, minced
- ½ tsp. paprika
- 8 oz. (230g) spinach
- ½ avocado

Directions:

Mash the garbanzo beans with a fork, leaving some whole. Mix in the turmeric and paprika, and season with salt and pepper.

Heat the oil in a pan over medium-high heat and sauté the onion and garlic for 2-3 minutes, until fragrant.

Add in the mashed garbanzo beans and cook for another 5 minutes, then transfer to a bowl, cover and set aside. Using the same pan, wilt the spinach, adding a tablespoon of water.

Once ready, divide the spinach between 2 bowls, top with the garbanzo beans and serve with avocado.

&

4. Vegan Frittata

My husband makes a Spanish frittata that was the first meal he ever made for me, so that dish has a special place in my heart. However, it uses eggs and butter, so I had to come up with a vegan version. I looked online, but many of the recipes were too particular, meaning you had to use specific ingredients, many of which are not available everywhere. I decided to adapt this, which uses tofu as the main ingredient, but I've listed the optional ingredients separately.

Like an omelet, the only limit is your imagination! And instead of oil, you're going to use vegetable broth to sauté the vegetables. This serves 6, but you can easily divide or multiply for the number of people you're serving. It's a great brunch idea.

Ingredients:

The Base:
- ¼ cup vegetable broth (see Vegan Basics) or use organic low-salt packaged broth
- 1 medium sweet onion, chopped
- 2 cloves of garlic, minced
- 14 ounces of firm tofu, drained
- 2 Tbsp. nutritional yeast
- ½ cup of water

Vegetable Choices: Mix and match to your heart's content

Original mixture:
- 12 oz. asparagus, tips only cut in ½-inch pieces
- 1 cup of sun-dried tomatoes, chopped
- 1 (14 ounces) can artichoke hearts in water, coarsely chopped

My favorites:

Spinach mixture:
- 1 cup finely chopped spinach
- 1 cup chopped mushrooms
- ½ tsp. (or more) rubbed thyme
- Salt and pepper to taste

Broccoli:
- 1 ½ cups finely chopped broccoli florets
- ½ cup finely chopped red pepper
- ½ to ¾ cup Vegan Mozzarella (in Vegan Basics)

Directions:

Preheat the oven to 400°F (200°C). Grease a springform pan (unless you have a cast iron pan that can go in the oven. In that case, use the cast iron pan for the sauté as well, but you will need to put a little oil in the bottom to make it easier to remove the frittata later.)

Heat the broth in a medium sauté pan. Add the onion and garlic. Stir in the vegetables. Cook for 3-4 minutes.

While that's cooking, blend the tofu, water, and nutritional yeast in a food processor until smooth.

Add the mixture to the saucepan with the vegetables.

Season with salt and pepper or any other spices you like, to taste.

Spoon into a springform pan or leave in the cast iron skillet. Bake for about 30-40 minutes.

Cut into wedges and serve.

&

5. **Buckwheat Apple Muesli** (despite its name, buckwheat is not a grain – it is a berry)

Ingredients:

- 3 ½ oz. (or 100 g.) buckwheat soaked for 1 hour or until tender
- 1 large apple chopped (preferably organic)
- ½ cup unsweetened, organic apple juice or enough so it will blend to a smooth consistency
- ½ tsp. ground cinnamon
- 2 Tbsp. maple syrup to taste

Garnish:

- dried cranberries or raisins
- coconut yogurt or shredded coconut
- toasted almonds or toasted buckwheat

Directions:

Once the buckwheat is tender (you can squish the grains between your fingers), drain it into a fine mesh sieve and rinse under a tap.

Place the sieve over a bowl and leave any excess water to drain while you prepare the remaining ingredients.

Place the chopped apple, apple juice, cinnamon, and 1 tablespoon of the maple syrup into a blender.

Add the drained buckwheat and blend until smooth, adding more apple juice as needed to assist with the blending.

Taste and add more maple syrup as needed.

Divide the muesli between 2 or 3 bowls and top with garnishes.

☟

6. Ginger Spiced Tofu Pancakes

Ingredients:

- 200 g. (approximately 1 ½ cups) garbanzo bean flour*
- 5.25 oz. (150 g.) soft tofu
- 1 Tbsp. ginger
- 1 onion, finely diced
- 1 carrot, grated
- 1 red or green pepper, finely diced
- 2 Tbsp. fresh cilantro, chopped
- Salt and pepper to taste
- 2 Tbsp. avocado or coconut oil

Directions:

Mix together the garbanzo bean flour, salt, and pepper in a large bowl.

Add the remaining ingredients except for half of the chopped cilantro and stir until the mixture is well combined.

Heat a safe non-stick or cast-iron pan to medium heat and scoop the pancake mixture into the pan in your desired size. There are usually 8 pancakes in this recipe.

Cook gently, flipping occasionally until golden-brown.

Sprinkle with cilantro and serve immediately. Serve with a hot chili sauce for extra flavor.

> ** Because the weight of different brands of garbanzo bean flour can have different volumes, it is best to weigh the flour for this recipe.*

7. Sweet Potato Anti-Inflammatory Muffins

I make these often. They are delicious, grain-free, anti-inflammatory, and they freeze well. A great light breakfast with a cup of coffee or tea.

Ingredients:

- 1 cup packed sweet potato puree – approximately one medium sweet potato
  (see Note below)
- 3 Tbsp. ground flaxseed left to sit in ½ cup of water for ten minutes
- 2 Tbsp. olive oil
- ¾ cup coconut milk (or almond or hemp milk, although coconut tastes best)
- ½ cup real maple syrup
- 1 cup brown rice flour
- ¼ cup coconut flour
- 1 Tbsp. ground cinnamon
- 1 Tbsp. baking powder
- 1 tsp. ground turmeric
- 1 tsp. ground ginger
- ½ tsp. salt
- ⅛ tsp. ground cloves
- ⅛ tsp. ground nutmeg

Directions:

Bake or boil the sweet potato. See the Note below regarding quantity.

After the potato has cooled a bit, process it until it turns into a puree. I use the food processor because it blends much better in the batter, but you can also just mash with a fork or potato masher.

Preheat oven to 400°F (200°C).

Oil a 12-count muffin tray or line with silicon baking cups.

Prepare the flaxseed mixture and set aside.

Add the coconut milk, maple syrup, olive oil, and flaxseed mixture to the sweet potato.

Blend until the mixture reaches a smooth consistency.

Sift the flours into a separate bowl and add all the dry ingredients.

Add combined dry ingredients to the potato mixture and stir until thoroughly combined.

Fill prepared muffin tray with batter so that each portion is approximately 2/3 full.

Bake 30 - 35 minutes. Don't over-bake, these muffins can get dry.

Cool on a rack for at least 5 minutes before enjoying.

* Note: I always cook several sweet potatoes at a time because I use them so much. It's easier on me and the environment to cook them in batches and have several ready in the fridge all the time. Cooked sweet potatoes also freeze well, so cook up a bunch!

I usually double this recipe, so I can freeze the muffins for convenience. They're so good!

Lunches

1. NotEgg Salad

Garbanzo beans (chickpeas) are incredibly versatile and packed full of nutri-ents, so I use them a lot. They are also inexpensive, especially if you buy bags of the dried beans and cook them yourself. However, cans are much more convenient and you get the benefit of the aquafaba, which is the water you drain from the cans. If you go online, you'll fine endless suggestions for using aquafaba, including as an egg replacer.

Ingredients:

- 1 (15-ounce) can garbanzo beans, rinsed and drained (or use 1 ½ cups cooked from dried)
- 2 small or 1 large avocado
- Juice from a lime or ½ lemon
- ¼ cup chopped red or green onion
- ¼ cup chopped celery (about 2 stalks)
- ½ tsp. garlic powder
- ½ tsp. onion powder
- ½ tsp. turmeric
- ¼ tsp. salt
- ¼ tsp. pepper

Directions:

Rinse the garbanzo beans and mash them in a bowl.

Add the avocados and mash into the beans.

Add the spices, onion, and celery.

Mix well.

You can use this in wraps with lettuce or sprouts or wrap the filling in lettuce leaves. I love just putting some sprouts on cucumbers sliced lengthwise and spreading the filling over that. Top with a dash of paprika. Yum!

This is also easy to take to work with you. Keep the salad separate from the lettuce and cucumber (or if you decide to eat some kind of bread or wrap, keep those separate).

Add some chia, pumpkin, hemp, or sunflower seeds sprinkled on top for extra omega-3 and crunchy taste.

2. Bowl Lunches

These are among my favorite things to make because it's a great way to use up leftovers and ensure nothing goes to waste. For dressing, you can also put a nice big forkful of fermented cabbage or kimchi on top. Sauerkraut makes an excellent dressing! Or you can make this healthy dressing here:

Dressing:

- 1 cup tahini
- ½ cup lemon or lime juice
- 1 Tbsp. fresh dill, or if none is available, 1 tsp. dried OR use cilantro or parsley, whatever makes you happy

Mix thoroughly. This will last in the fridge for three or four days, depending on which herb you use.

Components of the bowls

One portion each of:

Rice or quinoa
Black or red or garbanzo or cannellini beans – whatever you might have left over from other dishes

Fresh kale or baby spinach or dandelion greens – anything leafy and green that is solid (not lettuce)

Finely sliced red onion or some chopped green onion

Mix it up and toss with dressing.

You can also sprinkle nuts or seeds on top for extra flavor – stick to a tablespoon or so to keep the fat in check.

3. Quinoa Tabbouleh

Ingredients:

- 1 cup (170g) quinoa
- 2 medium tomatoes, finely diced
- 1 small cucumber, finely diced
- 1 bell pepper, finely diced
- 1 red onion, finely diced
- ⅔ cup (15g) parsley, chopped
- ⅔ cup (15g) mint, chopped
- juice of 2 limes
- 2 Tbsp. olive oil

Directions:

Cook the quinoa according to instructions on the packaging. Once cooked, place in a large salad bowl.

Finely dice the vegetables and chop the fresh herbs, then add to the salad bowl.

Squeeze in the lime juice, drizzle with olive oil, and season to taste with salt and pepper. Mix everything well until combined.

Serve as a salad or side dish. Store covered and refrigerated for up to three days.

This is easily made ahead and can be lunch for a few days.

☙

4. **Green Beans and Cherry Tomato Salad**

Ingredients:

- 1 lb. (450g) green beans
- 1 cup (150g) cherry tomatoes

For the dressing:

- 1 clove garlic, minced
- ⅓ cup (15g) cilantro, chopped
- 2 Tbsp. lemon juice
- ¼ cup (60ml) olive oil

Directions:

Trim the stem end of the green beans. Bring water to a boil in a large pot and cook the beans for 3 minutes. Then drain and rinse with cold water, allowing them to cool completely.

Halve the cherry tomatoes and place in a salad bowl. Once beans are cool cut them in one to two-inch pieces and add to the salad bowl.

Make the dressing by placing the dressing ingredients in a food processor. Pulse until a smooth sauce has formed. Season to taste with salt and pepper.

Add the sauce to the green beans and tomatoes and mix well until coated. Serve immediately as a salad or side dish. Store covered in the fridge for 2-3 days.

☙

5. Potato and Sun-Dried Tomato Salad

Ingredients:

- 1 lb. (450g) baby potatoes
- ½ cup (90g) green olives, halved
- ½ cup (70g) sun-dried tomatoes, drained, roughly chopped
- 2 Tbsp. capers, drained
- handful chives, chopped
- 1 Tbsp. oil from sun-dried tomatoes
- 1 Tbsp. wholegrain mustard
- 1 Tbsp. apple cider vinegar

Directions:

Place the potatoes in a pot of salted water and bring to a boil, lower the heat and simmer for about 20 minutes. Once cooked, drain and rinse in cold water. Once slightly cooled, peel, halve, and place them in a bowl.

Add in the olives, sun-dried tomatoes, capers, and chives. Next, mix the oil from the tomatoes, mustard, and apple cider vinegar and drizzle over the salad. Season to taste with salt and pepper, mix well, and serve.

6. Curried Tofu Salad

Ingredients:

- 7 oz. (200g) tofu, drained, crumbled
- 2 celery sticks, chopped
- 1 small onion, diced
- ¼ cup (30g) almonds, chopped
- ¼ cup (30g) raisins
- 3 Tbsp. vegan mayonnaise
- 1 tsp. curry powder
- 1 Tbsp. dill, chopped

Directions:

Crumble the tofu into a bowl. Add in the rest of the ingredients, season with salt and pepper, and stir well to combine.

Store in the fridge for up to 4-5 days.

7. The Best Change-It-Up Broccoli Salad

Broccoli is one of the best foods you can eat for brain health, so I use it a lot. This salad base is excellent because it not only uses broccoli, it also incorporates garbanzo beans and nuts or seeds, so you are boosting the nutritional value with every bite.

For the Basic Salad: Ingredients

- 1 head of broccoli, finely chopped
- 1 can garbanzo beans (or 1 ½ cups cooked from dried)
- 1 cup shredded carrots
- 1 bunch chopped green onions

Variations to add:

- ½ cup toasted sliced almonds
- ½ cup chopped walnuts or pecans
- ½ cup sunflower or pumpkin seeds
- ½ to ¾ cup chopped fresh cilantro
- ½ cup dried cranberries or raisins

Dressing Options:

For a curry-flavored dressing:

- ¼ cup tahini
- Juice of ½ large lemon

- 1 clove garlic, minced
- 1 tsp. yellow curry powder
- ½ Tbsp. freshly grated ginger (or if you don't have – you can use ½ tsp. powdered)
- ½ tsp. ground turmeric
- ½ tsp. salt
- 1 or 2 tsp. maple syrup (if you like a little sweetness)
- Freshly ground black pepper
- 2 to 4 Tbsp. warm water, as necessary, to thin dressing

Whisk all the ingredients together and pour over salad – toss to mix.

For a simple lemon and oil dressing:

- ¼ tsp. fine sea salt
- 1 Tbsp. fresh-squeezed lemon juice
- ¼ cup cold-pressed, extra virgin olive oil

Combine the sea salt and lemon juice in a small jar with lid, shake vigorously to mix well. Add the olive oil.

Voila! A great basic dressing – you can add a little garlic powder or thyme or rosemary depending on your taste. A bit of Dijon mustard is also a great addition.

The dressing lasts about 3 days in the fridge.

Directions:

Mix your chosen salad ingredients in a large bowl and set aside.

This salad keeps well up to 5 days in the fridge, but if you plan on using it over more than a couple of days, add the nuts and seeds on serving day so that they stay crunchier.

Dinners

1. Broccoli Mushroom Curry and Beans

Ingredients:

- 1 small head broccoli
- 8 oz. sliced mushrooms – button or cremini, your choice
- 1 large onion, roughly chopped
- 4 cloves garlic, minced
- 2 tsp. curry
- 2 tsp. turmeric
- ¼ tsp. cumin
- ¼ tsp. pepper
- Salt to taste
- 1 to 2 Tbsp. rice vinegar (to taste)
- 1 cup cooked brown rice
- 1 cup cooked garbanzo beans (or one 15 oz. can if using canned)
- Olive or avocado oil – normally I prefer avocado for high heat, but you don't have to use high heat for this recipe.

Directions:

Cut the broccoli into small chunks – use the whole head, not just the florets! (No waste!) Make them small enough that they will sauté easily.

Put a couple of tablespoons of oil into the pan and heat it. Add the broccoli and gently sauté until just approaching tender. Remove from the pan.

Add a bit more oil and sauté the chopped onions 5 minutes or so until translucent.

Add the garlic, curry, turmeric, cumin, and pepper and sauté a couple of minutes more, until the spices become fragrant. (Notice all these brain-boosting spices!)

Add the broccoli, mix lightly, and add the mushrooms. Gently sauté, mixing continuously, until the mushrooms are just approaching done. Then add the brown rice and garbanzo beans, then the rice vinegar.

Stir constantly and heat on medium until everything is warm – taste test for salt and curry.

This dish is awesome on its own, but I often add a few slices of avocado on top for extra flavor and healthy fats to boost the bioavailability of the turmeric.

2. Brain-Boosting Black Beans, Quinoa, and Zucchini

This recipe was developed by me specifically to help boost the immune system, which is essential to a healthy brain. Extra bonus: It's amazingly easy!

Ingredients for Zucchini Base:

- 4 medium zucchini squash – I like two green and two yellow for color, but whatever you can find
- 2 medium ripe tomatoes
- 1 large or 2 small onions
- 3 to 4 cloves garlic
- 220 grams (8 oz.) thinly sliced mushrooms – any kind will do, and a mixture is even better
- 2 Tbsp. coconut oil for frying

Spices:

- 4 tsps. curry
- 2 Tbsp. turmeric
- 1 tsp. black pepper
- 2 Tbsp. ground ginger, or a good 1-inch piece of fresh ginger, grated
- 1 tsp. paprika (I like Hungarian but whatever you have – add more to taste)
- 1 lemon, juiced

For the Quinoa and Beans:

- 2 cups cooked quinoa
- 1 cup cooked black beans
- 1 to 1 ½ Tbsp. olive oil for flavoring mixture
- Salt to taste
- Lemon pepper or regular pepper – whatever you have, to taste

Directions:

If you're using dried beans, soak and cook them ahead of time. If using canned beans, one can is sufficient – you will just be adding them to the quinoa once it is cooked.

Cook the quinoa. It takes around 20 minutes so if you're a slow sous chef, cut up the veggies first. If you're speedy, cut them up after you start the quinoa. It takes about 20 minutes.

Cut up all the veggies. I cut the zucchini lengthwise, then halve them again and slice the quarters into ½-inch pieces. Tomatoes – into 8 pieces each or so. Cut the onion into slivers to soak up the spices and oil. Crush garlic and ginger if you are using fresh ginger. Thin slice the mushrooms.

Put the coconut oil in your wok or similar pan, heat it just to warm, then add the turmeric, curry, pepper, and paprika (and ginger if you're using dried). Stir up the spices with a wooden paddle or spoon until they are aromatic, then throw in the onions.

Cook over medium to medium-high heat, stirring often, for about 5 minutes until the onions are just heading to soft. Then add the garlic and if using fresh ginger, add that now. Mix well and continue stirring to release all the aromatics. You want the onions to be semi-soft.

Add the zucchini and continue stirring, until the zucchini is just bordering on tender. Add the tomatoes, stir a couple of times. Then add the mushrooms. Keep stirring and add salt to taste. Just before all the veggies are at your desired level of "doneness," add the lemon juice, also to taste.

I add just enough to brighten up the dish and lift all the spices, but this is a "to taste" thing.

I put any extra lemon juice in with the quinoa and black beans.

Now that the veggies are basically done, your quinoa should be ready. Add the beans to the quinoa along with the salt and pepper and olive oil. The remaining lemon juice can go in here if you like.

Mix well.

Serve the quinoa and rice on the bottom of flat soup-like bowls and cover with your veggies.

Served with a small green salad with purple onion, cucumber, lime, and cilantro, you have a high protein, nutrient-rich meal full of antioxidants and immune boosters.

&⟩

3. Veggie "Pasta" with Vegan "Alfredo" Sauce

Quick, easy, and incredibly delicious. Make zucchini spirals, spaghetti squash, or quinoa or chia pasta and top with this delicious sauce. Serve with a green salad and you have the perfect meal for any night of the week.

This sauce is great no matter what you put it on! Just have your veggies or pasta basically cooked when you start the sauce, as it is ready fast.

The "Alfredo" sauce Ingredients:

- 1 cup milk of choice
- ⅔ cup fully mashed avocado (160g)
- ¼ tsp. garlic powder
- ½ tsp. salt, or more to taste
- 2 tsp. olive oil or Vegan Butter (see Vegan Basics). This adds richness and helps the sauce adhere to pasta, but it can be omitted.

Directions:

Mix all ingredients together in a small saucepan, whisk until smooth. Heat until sauce thickens and begins to boil, then stir in the spiralized zucchini, spaghetti squash, or pasta and remove from the heat. Serve immediately, sprinkling with nutritional yeast.

ॐ

4. **Sesame Tempeh Stir-Fry** – this is a tasty way to incorporate more fermented foods.

Ingredients:

- 7 oz. (200g) tempeh, cut into cubes
- 1 Tbsp. olive oil
- 1 Tbsp. ginger, grated
- 2 cloves garlic, crushed
- 1 Tbsp. sesame oil
- 1 Tbsp. rice wine vinegar
- 3 Tbsp. tamari (or soy sauce)
- 2 Tbsp. maple syrup
- 2 carrots, chopped or cut into thin strips
- ½ broccoli head, florets
- 1 bell pepper, sliced
- 1 Tbsp. sesame seeds, to garnish
- spring onion or chives, to garnish
- 3 cups (585g), organic wild rice, cooked

Directions:

Heat the olive oil in a pan over medium-high heat and cook the tempeh for about 6 minutes, occasionally stirring until browned on each side.

In the meantime, prepare the sauce by mixing ginger, garlic, sesame oil, rice wine vinegar, tamari (or soy sauce), and maple syrup in a bowl.

Add half the sauce to the pan with the tempeh, mix until coated, then remove it from the pan and set it aside.

Add the carrots, broccoli, pepper, and remaining sauce to the pan and cook for about 5 minutes, or until veggies are tender.

Add in the tempeh and cook for another 3-5 minutes or until the vegetables are cooked through.

Once ready, serve with the organic wild rice, sesame seeds, and sliced spring onion or chives. You can substitute riced cauliflower for the rice.

5. Veggie and Tahini Bake – easy and delicious!

Ingredients:

- 1 onion, sliced
- 1 zucchini, sliced
- 1 red bell pepper, sliced
- 1 cup (265g) garbanzo beans, drained
- 1 Tbsp. olive oil
- 3 Tbsp. tahini
- 1 lemon, juice only
- 3 Tbsp. almond milk
- 1 Tbsp. sesame seeds
- handful coriander (cilantro), chopped

Directions:

Preheat oven to 375°F (190°C).

Place the chopped vegetables in a baking tray, drizzle with olive oil, and season with salt and pepper. Mix well and cook in the oven for 35 minutes or until vegetables are cooked.

In a small bowl, mix the tahini, lemon juice, milk, and sesame seeds, then set aside.

Once vegetables are cooked, mix them with the tahini sauce and serve with fresh coriander.

6. **Tempeh Bolognese** – more fermented goodness!

Ingredients:

- 8 oz. (225g) gluten-free/grain-free penne such as chia, quinoa, or garbanzo bean (chickpea) pasta
- 1 Tbsp. olive oil
- 3 cloves garlic, minced
- 1 medium onion, chopped
- 1 red bell pepper, chopped
- 7 oz. (200g) tempeh, crumbled
- 14 oz. (400g) can chopped tomatoes
- 2 Tbsp. tomato puree
- 1 Tbsp. apple cider vinegar
- 1 tsp. mixed herbs
- fresh basil, for serving

Directions:

Cook pasta according to instructions on the packaging.

Heat olive oil over medium-high heat in a large pan. Add garlic and onion and sauté until fragrant, for about 3-4 minutes. Add in bell pepper and crumbled tempeh and sauté for another 5 minutes.

Reduce heat to medium-low and add chopped tomatoes, tomato puree, vinegar, and mixed herbs – season with salt and pepper. Bring to boil and let it simmer for 5-6 minutes or until heated through.

To serve, divide pasta and Bolognese between plates and garnish with basil.

7. Mushroom Cauliflower Risotto

Ingredients:

- 2 Tbsp. olive oil
- 2 cloves garlic, minced
- 1 cup mushrooms, roughly chopped
- 1 cup unsweetened coconut milk or ½ cup unsweetened coconut cream
- ⅓ cup low-sodium vegetable broth (see Vegan Basics for recipe or use from a carton)
- ½ cup Vegan Parmesan (see Vegan Basics for recipe)
- 2 cups riced cauliflower
- salt and pepper to taste

Directions:

In a safe non-stick (or cast iron) skillet, on medium-high heat, add olive oil and garlic. Cook for about 1-2 minutes.

Add the mushrooms. Cook for about 3-5 minutes.

Add the riced cauliflower. Cook for another 2-3 minutes, stirring frequently. Careful not to let it burn!

Add coconut milk (or cream), vegetable broth, and Vegan Parmesan. Stir to combine.

Reduce heat to low, then cover and let it simmer for about 15 minutes, until desired creamy consistency.

Serve immediately. (I like to add a side salad of tomatoes and green onions with a tiny bit of lemon juice, salt, and pepper – adds color and brightens the taste.)

8. Portobello Mushrooms Stuffed with Broccoli and Spinach

Ingredients:

For mushrooms and stuffing:
- 2 large portobello mushrooms
- ½ cup cooked or canned black beans
- 2 cups finely chopped broccoli florets
- 1 cup finely chopped spinach
- 3 garlic cloves, crushed
- ½ medium onion, finely chopped
- 1 tsp. ground rosemary
- 1 tsp. rubbed thyme
- Olive oil
- Salt and pepper

For sauce to go in stuffing:
Use the recipe for the **Vegan "Alfredo" Sauce** in #3 above.

Directions:

Preheat oven to 350°F (175°C).

Scoop the fins off the mushrooms and remove stems as you are going to be stuffing them. Brush with olive oil, bake until just tender while you are making the filling.

Make the **Vegan "Alfredo" Sauce**.

Lightly sauté the onion and garlic.

Mix all veggies, including the chopped up mushroom stems, spices, and beans, in a large bowl, add the Alfredo sauce, and mix well.

Stuff the partially cooked mushrooms with the filling (it's okay to load them up!). Bake 15 to 20 minutes more until tender – will depend on the size of the mushrooms and how much you filled them.

Serve with a fresh salad.

&

9. Lentil Shepherd's Pie

Ingredients:

- 1 Tbsp. olive oil
- 1 cup chopped leeks (can substitute white onion)
- 1 cup chopped carrots
- 1 cup chopped celery
- 3 garlic cloves, chopped
- 1 cup green (or brown) lentils
- 3 cups vegetable broth (see in Vegan Basics, or purchase organic, low salt)

You may need up to 4 cups.
- 2 bay leaves
- 1 bundle fresh thyme – you can substitute with 2 tsp. dried thyme
- 1 stem fresh rosemary – you can substitute with 1 tsp. dried rosemary
- 3 Tbsp. tomato paste
- 2 pounds potatoes, chopped into 1" pieces (See Note below.)
- 1 tsp. salt
- ½ to ¾ cup unsweetened almond or hemp milk
- ¼ cup Vegan Butter, melted (See Vegan Basics)
- 1 Tbsp. chopped parsley
- 1 cup frozen peas

Directions:

Heat the olive oil in a large wide pan (like a Dutch oven) over medium heat.

Add the onion, carrots, celery and a pinch of salt and freshly ground pepper. Cook for 10 minutes until vegetables are soft and tender.

Add in the garlic, lentils, vegetable broth, bay leaves, thyme, rosemary and bring to a boil.

Reduce heat to a low, cover and simmer for 30-35 minutes until lentils are tender.

Stir every 5 minutes or so to ensure the vegetables don't stick to the bottom of the pan. You may need to add more vegetable broth/water: start with 3 cups broth and go from there, up to 4 cups.

Once lentils are cooked, whisk in the tomato paste.

While the lentils are cooking, make the potatoes. Place the potatoes in a medium saucepan and cover by 1-inch with water. Stir in the salt and bring water to a boil. Reduce heat to medium and simmer potatoes until they are fork tender, about 15 minutes.

Drain the water from the potatoes and mash them thoroughly with milk and butter while they are still hot.

Season to taste with salt and freshly ground pepper.

Remove the bay leaves, thyme bundle, rosemary and discard from the lentil mixture and stir in the peas.

Preheat the broiler. Transfer the lentil mixture to a 9×13 baking dish. Spread the mashed potatoes over the lentils in an even layer. Place the baking dish under the preheated broiler and broil until the potatoes are golden brown and crispy, about 5 minutes.

Remove from oven and serve.

Note: I have made this several times with mashed sweet potatoes. The dish tastes more complex and a bit richer, so this is definitely something to consider.

Vegan Basics

There are many recipes for all of these online, but these are what I use because we don't have access to cashews here, which is a common ingredient for vegan cheese and butter online. Also, even if you're in North America, cashews can be expensive AND there are some serious ethical considerations regarding processing.

1. Vegan Butter

Ingredients:

- ⅓ cup unsweetened almond or hemp milk
- 1 tsp. apple cider vinegar
- 1 cup (melted or liquid) refined coconut oil (refined so you don't taste the coconut in the butter)
- 2 Tbsp. avocado or hemp oil
- 1 tsp. nutritional yeast
- ½ tsp. pink salt

Directions:

Pour the liquid coconut oil and hemp or avocado oil in a blender.

In a separate measuring cup, mix the hemp milk and apple cider vinegar. They will curdle slightly.

Pour this mixture into the blender, then add nutritional yeast and salt.

Process until very smooth.

Store in a small glass dish in the refrigerator. It will solidify in a couple of hours.

Can be stored for 2 weeks or so in the fridge. If you need longer than that to use it up, split the recipe in half and freeze half. It freezes well.

2. Vegan Mozzarella

Ingredients:

- Soak 1 tsp. psyllium husk with 1 Tbsp. water
- ⅓ cup sunflower seeds (rinsed and then soaked in warm water at least 2 hours)
- 1 ¼ cups water
- 4 Tbsp. nutritional yeast
- 2 Tbsp. cornstarch
- 2 tsp. pink salt
- 1 Tbsp. white vinegar
- Scant ¼ cup coconut oil (refined)
- 1 Tbsp. agar (optional – this is to make the cheese firmer for slicing)

Directions:

Mix everything together in high-speed blender.

Pour into a pan and whisk continuously as you cook the mixture over medium heat.

Cheese is done when it becomes stringy like melted mozzarella.

Store in a glass container in the refrigerator up to 2 weeks.

3. Vegan Parmesan

Ingredients:

- ⅓ cup raw hemp or pumpkin seeds or almonds or walnuts or a combination of these
- ¼ cup nutritional yeast
- 1 Tbsp. potato starch or rice flour (to keep the product drier)

- ½ tsp. salt
- ¼ tsp. garlic powder

Optional:
- ⅛ tsp. dry mustard powder

Directions:

Add the seeds and/or nuts with all other ingredients to a blender jar.

Pulse in 5-second increments until it reaches a sandy texture.

Store in an airtight container at room temperature for 2 weeks or in the refrigerator for up to 2 months.

&

4. **Vegetable Stock – really important to use organic vegetables for this recipe if at all possible**

Ingredients:

- 1 large brown onion
- 4 ribs celery
- 5 medium carrots
- 6 cloves garlic
- 3 Tbsp. olive oil
- 1 Tbsp. sea salt
- ½ Tbsp. peppercorns
- 12 cups water

Directions:

Wash and roughly chop the vegetables. Better not to peel as you keep more of the beneficial nutrients.

Crush and peel the garlic cloves.

In a large stock pot, heat the olive oil and sauté the vegetables for 5 minutes.

Add the water, stir in the salt and peppercorns.

Bring all to a boil, then reduce to a gentle simmer for 1 hour.

Separate the broth from the vegetables, then remove the majority of peppercorns from the vegetables. If you like a hearty stock, mix batches of the stock with the vegetables in a high-speed blender. When I make this recipe, I make half as a "heavy" stock, and leave the other half "light."

The broth freezes easily either way.

If I don't blend and use all of the vegetables in the broth because I want a light broth, I take whatever is left and mix it with rice or quinoa the next day and spice it up with turmeric and curry and whatever else I feel like because I cannot stand throwing out food!

Note: If you have leftover fresh herbs like rosemary or thyme, you can use them up here.

5. Coconut Milk Yogurt

You need a crock pot or Instant Pot for this recipe – and this is fussy and takes time and planning. I do this because it is impossible to get pure coconut milk yogurt here where I live in Ecuador. But I thought I would offer it in case you are in an area where it is hard to find plant-based yogurts. This also works for soy milk, and I'm told it is thicker, although I do not eat much soy.

Making this is a bit of a process because it usually takes a couple of batches to get it really thick. I am in Ecuador, so I can make my own coconut milk as thick as I like it using fresh coconut flesh and coconut water (in a high-speed blender). But if you're somewhere where coconut milk is mostly sold in cans, you can certainly use that. Or coconut cream is even better so that the yogurt will be thicker.

Ingredients:

- 4 cups coconut cream if possible (milk will do)
- 1 capsule of a good probiotic (the more strains the better)

OR 1 container of plain coconut yogurt from the store (starter)

Directions:

Place the 4 cups of coconut milk in the crockpot and turn it on low. Let sit for 2.5 hours.

When the 2.5 hours are up, turn the crockpot off and let it sit for 2 hours.

When the 2 hours are up, take 1 cup of the warm milk or cream out of the crockpot and mix it with the starter OR empty the contents of the probiotic capsule into the cup and mix very well. If you're using a starter yogurt, leave it out for a couple of hours so it is not cold when you mix it up with the warm milk from the crock pot.

Put the mixture back in the crockpot and take the vessel out of the heating element, wrap in a heavy towel, and either put it in a cupboard or inside the oven (that is not turned on) for 8 to 10 hours. This is where the magic happens.

I started off with 9 hours and it was a bit too much so I now only do it for 8 hours, but it kind of depends on how "sour" you like your yogurt to taste.

After the 8 or 9 or 10 hours – take it out of wherever you've let it sit and put the vessel in the fridge to cool.

If you're using probiotics it will take a few batches to get thicker yogurt. But from now on you don't have to use the probiotics. You are going to save ½ cup of the yogurt you've made to use for your next batch.

It will be runny at first. I use it for smoothies, but if you want to have it thicker, just strain it so that the heavier/thicker batch is separated from the runnier product.

For the Vegan Tzatziki Sauce recipe in this book, you will want a thicker yogurt, so you might just want to use a plain vegan yogurt from the store.

6. Lentil Tortillas

Ingredients:

- ¾ cup red lentils
- 1 ¼ cup filtered water
- ¼ tsp. sea or pink salt

Directions:

Rinse and drain the lentils well. Soak them in the filtered water for at least 3 hours.

Blend the soaked lentils together with the soaking water, salt, and optional flavorings until smooth. I usually have to add a little more water to make the batter more like pancake batter, which is what you're aiming for.

Heat a safe non-stick pan to medium heat. Do not add oil.

Measure about 1/4 cup of the batter to the pan and spread it evenly in a circle to about the thickness of a crepe or a little more. Not too thin, or it won't stand up to all the goodies you can place inside.

Cook until the top begins to harden, then carefully flip and cook the other side until slightly browned. It takes about 2 minutes per tortilla.

They can be frozen, but they never last long enough in our house to save them that way. To reheat, use the pan – don't microwave.

Optional ingredients: Black pepper, garlic or onion powder - about ¼ tsp.

7. Yucca Flour Tortillas

Ingredients:

- 1 ½ cups yucca flour (make sure it's not tapioca flour – that doesn't work, and there are some brands of cassava or yucca flour that do not work. Because I'm in Ecuador, I don't know N. American or European brands, so you may have to do some experimentation)
- ½ tsp. salt
- ⅛ tsp. garlic or onion powder
- ¼ cup olive or avocado oil
- ¾ cup warm water plus more if needed

Directions:

Whisk together the flour, salt, and garlic or onion powder. Be sure they're thoroughly mixed.

Add oil and ½ cup of the warm water to start. Knead with your hands and check the consistency – it should be like bread dough. If you need more water, add a bit at a time and knead again until thoroughly mixed.

Divide the dough into 8 equal portions and roll them into balls.

Roll each ball with a rolling pin between two pieces of parchment paper or silicone mats. You want them to be about ⅛-inch thick and about 5 inches in diameter.

If you have a tortilla press, this is the time to use it.

Heat a safe non-stick skillet or griddle over medium-high heat. Do not add oil.

Cook each tortilla for 1-2 minutes per side, or until it begins to bubble.

Serve warm with your favorite ingredients.

These can be frozen – just put sheets of parchment paper between them in a freezer lock bag so you can take out just one or two at a time.

Note that with some brands of the yucca or cassava flour you may not end up with bread-like dough. However, even if it's not perfect dough, you can make the tortillas by ladling the mixture like pancake dough into the pan. I've had to do it a few different ways depending on the flour available, and while the process can be a little frustrating, they always taste great.

Desserts and Sweet Energy Treats

It is hard to give up sugar when you first start, but if you have something that takes its place, like healthy cacao in delicious desserts, it is a lot easier. Enjoy!

1. Chocolate Zucchini Bread

Ingredients:

- 1 ½ cups grated zucchini
- 2 Tbsp. ground flax seeds in 6 Tbsp. water (egg replacement)
- 1 ¼ cup almond flour (you can also use garbanzo bean flour, but it has a stronger taste)
- ⅓ cup cacao powder
- 1 tsp. baking soda
- pinch of salt
- ¾ cup brown sugar or coconut sugar
- ½ cup Vegan Butter or coconut oil, melted
- ¼ cup non-dairy milk unsweetened
- 1 tsp. of vanilla extract

Directions:

Grate the zucchini.

Combine the ground flax seeds and water in a small bowl and whisk until fully incorporated. Set aside to thicken.

Preheat oven to 350°F (175°C). Line or grease a standard 8.5" x 4.5" loaf pan.

Sift together the flour, cocoa powder, baking soda, and salt in a large bowl. Set aside.

In a medium bowl, mix together the sugar, coconut oil, or Vegan Butter, milk, and vanilla until well combined. Add the flax mixture and mix again.

Combine all ingredients in the large bowl. Fold in the zucchini. (If you wanted to add raw cacao nibs here, this would be the time to do it. One-half cup or so adds a little dimension to the recipe.)

Transfer the batter to the baking pan and bake for 50 minutes, or until a toothpick inserted into the center of the loaf comes out clean.

Cool the loaf before removing it from the pan.

ॐ

2. Banana "Ice Cream"

This is a great way to use up bananas that are getting overripe.

Peel, cut them up in chunks, and freeze on a cookie sheet. Then place them in a freezer bag for use in smoothies or this recipe.

When you're ready for ice cream, take out as many as you need, let them defrost just a bit, then process in the food processor until they are the consistency you like. Add some fresh or frozen fruit, cacao, or coconut, and process again until smooth.

Refreeze for a while, or if you like soft-serve, eat right out of the food processor. (That's my favorite!)

All the nutrients of bananas and whatever fruit you like and no simple sugars or dairy or anything processed. The perfect answer for a sweet craving!

ॐ

3. Avocado-Banana Chocolate Pudding

Ingredients:

- 3 bananas, peeled and cut into pieces (medium-ripe)
- 1 ½ medium-ripe avocados, pitted and peeled
- ⅔ cup coconut milk

- 6 Tbsp. unsweetened cocoa powder
- ⅔ tsp. pure vanilla extract
- ¼ tsp. freshly ground cinnamon
- ¼ tsp. sea salt
- Dried coconut shavings

Directions:

Save a few small pieces of the banana to garnish the pudding. Put the rest in a food processor, add the avocado and coconut milk, and process until smooth.

Add cocoa powder, vanilla extract, cinnamon, and sea salt to food processor. Mix until creamy.

If the mixture is too thick, add more coconut milk until you achieve the desired texture.

Place in an airtight container to cool down.

Serve topped with the sliced banana and dried coconut shavings.

4. Chia Seed Pudding

- 3-4 Tbsp. chia seeds
- 1 cup milk (I like unsweetened coconut, almond, or cashew milk)
- ½ Tbsp. maple syrup
- ¼ tsp. vanilla (optional) or
- ¼ tsp. cinnamon (optional)
- Toppings of choice: fresh berries or other fruit, nut butter, etc.

Directions:

In a jar with a tight-fitting lid, stir together chia seeds, milk, maple syrup, and vanilla or cinnamon, if using. Shake the mixture to combine everything.

Once the mixture is well combined, let it sit for 5 minutes, then give it another shake to break up any clumps of seeds. Cover and put the mixture in the fridge to set for 2 hours or overnight. If it is not thick enough when you take it out, just add more chia seeds (about 1 tablespoon), stir, and refrigerate for another 30 minutes or so.

Chia pudding can be stored for up to 5-7 days in an airtight container in the refrigerator.

❧

5. Energy Balls

Ingredients:

- 1 cup (120g) dates, stones removed
- ¾ cup (60g) almond meal
- ½ cup (30g) desiccated coconut
- 2 Tbsp. chia seeds
- 2 Tbsp. coconut oil, melted
- 1 Tbsp. natural peanut butter

Directions:

Place all ingredients in a high-speed blender or food processor and blitz until everything is well combined and chopped to small pieces.

Using your hands, form 10 balls about the size of a walnut. Place them in the fridge to chill for at least 1 hour so that they become more solid.

Store in the fridge in an airtight container for up to 2 weeks.

❧

6. Lemon and Berry "Cheese"cake – With coconut, walnuts, dates, and chia seeds, it just doesn't get much better for your brain than this!

Ingredients:

For the crust:
- ½ cup (40g) desiccated coconut
- 1 cup (100g) walnuts, chopped
- 12 medjool dates
- pinch of salt

For the lemon layer:
- 2 cups (230g) cashews, soaked for 4 hours or overnight
- 1 cup (240ml) coconut cream
- 4 Tbsp. coconut oil, soft
- ½ cup (120ml) maple syrup
- zest of 1 lemon
- juice of 1 lemon juice
- pinch of salt

For the berry layer:
- 1 cup (150g) frozen red berries
- 2 Tbsp. chia seeds
- 2 Tbsp. lemon juice
- 2 Tbsp. maple syrup

Directions:

Place all the crust ingredients into a food processor and blitz until sticky paste forms. Transfer the crust into a cake tin or springform pan and press evenly to form the bottom layer. Place the tin in the freezer while you make the other layers.

Drain the cashews and pat dry with a kitchen towel. Place all the lemon-layer ingredients in a food processor and puree until smooth. Spread over the crust and return to the freezer.

Prepare the last berry layer. Place all ingredients in the food processor and puree until smooth. Spread over the top of the cheesecake only when the lemon layer has set completely. Garnish with additional berries (optional). Return to the freezer and freeze until set.

Remove the cheesecake from the freezer for about 20 minutes before serving.

7. Vegan Chocolate Brownies

Ingredients:

- 8 oz. (220g) 70% or greater dark chocolate, chopped
- 3 Tbsp. coconut oil
- 2 ripe avocados
- 1 cup (200g) coconut palm sugar
- 2 flax eggs*
- 1 tsp. vanilla extract
- ¾ cup (75g) almond meal
- ¼ cup (30g) unsweetened cocoa powder
- ½ tsp. baking powder
- ½ tsp. sea salt
- ½ cup (50g) walnuts, chopped

  HOW TO MAKE A FLAX EGG:
  To make one flax egg, mix 1 Tbsp. flaxseed meal and 2 ½ Tbsp.
  water. Let it rest for 5 mins to thicken.

Directions:

Preheat oven to 350°F (175°C).

Line an 8x8-inch baking pan with baking paper.

Place the coconut oil and chopped chocolate in a medium-sized heatproof bowl. Place the bowl over a pot of lightly simmering water. Stir the chocolate and coconut oil until they are completely melted.

In a large bowl, mash avocado and then stir in the chocolate mixture. Whisk in the sugar, then add in the flax eggs and vanilla extract, mix well.

Add in the cocoa powder, almond meal, baking powder, and salt, mixing until just combined (do not overmix).

Stir in chopped walnuts.

Spread the batter into the prepared baking tin and place it in the middle of the oven. Bake for about 25 to 30 minutes until the middle is set.

Let completely cool on a rack and cut into 12 squares.

Salads

I'm a big fan of salads that last a couple of days, because it's great to be able to "cook once, eat twice." Many of these fit that description and can be used for lunches and/or dinners.

1.   Fiesta Black Bean and Quinoa Salad

Ingredients: (proportions are not as important as variety – so whatever you like in the way of balance). This one lasts at least 3 days so is great for lunches. Very filling!

- Finely chopped celery
- Scallions
- Bell pepper
- Cucumber
- Spinach
- Cherry tomatoes
- 1 can black beans
- 1 ½ cups or so cooked quinoa
- 1 ½ cups or so cooked sweet corn

Season the whole mixture with your choice of:

- Crushed garlic
- Chili powder
- Cumin
- Cayenne pepper (if you like lots of spice)
- Pinch of salt

Add fresh-squeezed lime juice and optionally a small drizzle of olive oil, or substitute lime juice with lemon juice or cider vinegar.

Keeps well in the fridge for three days.

&

2. Garbanzo Bean Salad with Orange Miso Dressing

Ingredients:

- 12 cherry tomatoes, halved
- 4 green onions, sliced
- ½ cup dry quinoa
- 1 ½ cups low-sodium garbanzo beans (chickpeas), cooked or canned and rinsed
- 3 Tbsp. fresh cilantro
- ¼ cup fresh orange juice (juice of 2 oranges)
- ¼ cup seasoned rice vinegar
- 2 tsp. white or yellow miso
- 1 Tbsp. maple syrup or agave nectar
- 1 clove garlic, grated or minced
- 1 tsp. ginger, grated or minced
- 2 tsp. black sesame seeds

Directions:

Combine the tomatoes, onions, cooked quinoa, garbanzo beans, and fresh cilantro in a large bowl.

In a small bowl, thoroughly whisk the orange juice, rice vinegar, miso, maple syrup or agave nectar, garlic, ginger, and sesame seeds to make the dressing.

Pour the dressing into the larger bowl and toss all the salad ingredients together.

Instructions for quinoa:

Place 1 part quinoa to 2 parts water (for example: 1 cup quinoa to 2 cups water) in a saucepan and bring to a boil. Reduce to a simmer, cover, and cook until all the water is absorbed (about 15 minutes). You will know that the quinoa is done when all the grains have turned from white to transparent, and the spiral-like germ has separated. Wait for it to cool to add to the recipe. You could also substitute 1 cup of frozen, thawed quinoa for a precooked option.

3. Chopped Thai Garbanzo Bean Salad with Peanut Curry Dressing

Red cabbage and carrots are powerhouse veggies, and the spices in this dressing are all awesome anti-inflammatory nutrients, so enjoy often! This makes a great lunch because the cabbage and carrots hold up well with the dressing.

Ingredients:

For the salad:
- 1 red bell pepper, diced
- 1 cup shredded carrots
- 2 cups shredded red cabbage
- 1 (15 ounce) can garbanzo beans, rinsed and drained
- ½ cup cilantro, finely chopped
- ¼ cup finely chopped green onion
- ½ jalapeño, seeded and diced

For the curry peanut butter dressing:
- 2 Tbsp. peanut butter
- ½ Tbsp. freshly grated ginger
- 1 clove garlic, minced
- 1 tsp. apple cider vinegar
- 1 tsp. yellow curry powder
- ¼ tsp. red cayenne pepper
- ¼ tsp. ground turmeric
- Salt and freshly ground black pepper, to taste
- 2-3 Tbsp. warm water, to thin dressing

Extra cilantro for garnish

Directions:

Dressing: In a small bowl, mix together peanut butter, ginger, garlic, apple cider vinegar, curry powder, cayenne pepper, and turmeric. Add water to thin if necessary.

Salad: In a large bowl, mix all ingredients then add dressing and mix well to combine.

Garnish with cilantro.

&

4. Wild Rice, Tomato, and Arugula Salad

Ingredients:

- 1 cup (185g) wild rice
- ½ cup roasted peppers, drained, chopped
- ¼ cup (30g) roasted almonds, chopped
- 1 cup (150g) cherry tomatoes, halved
- 2 oz. (60g) arugula
- 1 Tbsp. balsamic vinegar
- 1 Tbsp. olive oil
- ½ tsp. chili flakes

Directions:

Cook the rice according to instructions on the packaging. Once cooked, place in a large bowl.

Add in the peppers, almonds, tomatoes, and arugula. Drizzle with vinegar and oil, add chili flakes, season to taste with salt and pepper, and mix until well combined, before serving.

&

5. Cleansing Kale Salad

Ingredients:

For the dressing:
- ½ cup of lemon juice

- ½ cup of olive oil
- 1 clove of garlic (minced)
- 1 tsp. fresh ginger (minced)
- 1 tsp. rosemary
- 1 tsp. maple syrup or equivalent of Stevia. (I skip it, but you might like the sweetness)
- A pinch of cayenne
- 1 Tbsp. salt

For the salad:
- 2 cups kale (chopped)
- 2 cups red cabbage (shredded)
- 2 cups broccoli (chopped)
- 2 carrots (shredded)
- 1 bell pepper (diced)
- 2 avocados (diced)
- ½ cup fresh parsley (chopped)
- 1 cup walnuts
- 1 Tbsp. sesame seeds

Directions:

Add all dressing ingredients to a medium-sized blender and process until the contents are fully integrated.

Slice up all the veggies and herbs per the instructions above.

Put everything into a salad bowl and toss it together.

Soups and Stews

For a whole-foods, plant-based lifestyle, the sheer number and range of soups and stews is enough to keep you eating well for years without repeating any recipe twice. I have chosen my favorites, based on their nutritional content and for the ingredients that are particularly powerful brain foods.

1. Vegan Mushroom Soup

Ingredients:

- 2 Tbsp. olive oil
- 1 large onion, diced
- 4 cloves garlic, minced
- 2 lbs. cremini or white mushroom (or mixed), sliced
- ½ cup dry red vegan wine (you can also use white) (OPTIONAL)
- 1 Tbsp. fresh thyme. If you don't have fresh, use 1 ½ tsp. dried thyme.
- 4 cups vegetable broth (See the recipe in Vegan Basics)
- 1 ½ cups almond or coconut milk
  Salt and pepper to taste

Optional: 5 Tbsp. cornstarch (organic if possible) in ⅓ cup cool water to thicken

Directions:

Sauté the onions and garlic approximately 5 minutes, until just tender and fragrant.

Add the mushrooms, wine, and thyme, cook another 5 minutes.

Add the broth, bring to a boil.

Cover and reduce heat, simmer for 15 minutes. Add the milk and cook 5 minutes more.

Optional: If you like a thicker soup, you can mix the cornstarch with the cool water in a separate cup and add to the mixture. It's like making gravy, so if you need to add more to make the soup thicker to your taste, adjust accordingly. Remove from heat and season with salt and pepper.

2. Simple Cauliflower Soup with Garlic and Rosemary

Ingredients:

- 6 cups water
- 1 large head of cauliflower cut into florets
- 1 onion, chopped
- 4 large cloves of garlic, minced
- 1 Tbsp. fresh rosemary OR dried rosemary, minced
- 1 tsp. sea salt
- 1 tsp. black pepper
- ½ bunch fresh parsley
- 1 Tbsp. extra virgin olive oil

Directions:

Add water and cauliflower florets to a large soup pot.

Add onion, garlic, rosemary, sea salt, and black pepper.

Simmer on medium-high heat for about 15 minutes. The cauliflower should be soft.

Carefully blend the hot mixture in batches using a blender or an immersion blender.

Taste for salt. Top with fresh parsley and olive oil before serving.

3. Moroccan Carrot Black Pepper Turmeric Soup – This is an anti-inflammatory powerhouse!

Ingredients:

- 2 Tbsp. Vegan Butter (see Vegan Basics) or avocado oil
- 1 cup chopped organic yellow onion
- 1 lb. large organic carrots, cut in ½-inch dices (about 2 ⅔ cups)
- 2 ½ cups Vegetable Stock (See recipe in Vegan Basics)
- 2 minced garlic cloves (or more to taste)
- 2 tsp. turmeric
- 1 ½ tsp. cumin seeds – finely ground
- 1 Tbsp. honey (if you're not 100% vegan) or maple syrup
- 1 Tbsp. fresh lemon juice
- ⅛ tsp. allspice
- Salt and fresh cracked black pepper (to taste)

Directions:

Melt butter or use avocado oil in a large saucepan over medium-high heat.

Add onion; sauté for 2 minutes. Mix in carrots and broth.

Bring to boil. Reduce heat, cover, and simmer until carrots are very tender, about 20 minutes.

Stir cumin seeds in a small skillet over medium-high heat until fragrant, about 4-5 minutes. Then finely grind in a spice mill or coffee grinder dedicated to spices.

Remove soup from heat. Puree in batches in a blender until smooth. Return to saucepan.

Whisk in honey or maple syrup, lemon juice, and allspice. Season with salt and pepper.

Ladle soup into bowl. Sprinkle with toasted cumin. Serve.

4. Herb and Spice Power Vegetable Soup

The turmeric and black pepper, garlic, and ginger are powerful anti-inflammatories and antibacterials. Add the rosemary and sage that are so good for memory and learning, and you have a powerful soup that is also good if you're feeling a bit under the weather.

Ingredients:

- 1 ½ tsp. turmeric
- ½ tsp. black pepper
- 1 tsp. rosemary
- 1 tsp. thyme
- 1 tsp. sage
- 1 tsp. basil
- 1 bay leaf
- 3 cloves garlic
- Fresh ginger measured to your liking
- ½ large onion, diced
- 2 large carrots, chopped
- 2 medium to large zucchini, chopped
- 7 cremini mushrooms, quartered
- 3 medium potatoes, chopped
- 1 bunch kale
- Pink salt (to taste)

Directions:

Sauté onions, garlic, and ginger until fragrant.

Add mushrooms, carrots, and zucchini until soft enough to pierce with a fork.

Cover all vegetables with water and bring to a boil.

Add all herbs.

Add potatoes, cover, and allow to boil for 30 minutes.

Add kale, cover, and boil for 10 minutes.

Salt to taste.

☙

5. Cauliflower with Turmeric and Garlic Soup

Ingredients:

- 1 bulb garlic, roasted
- 3 Tbsp. olive oil
- 1 medium onion (chopped)
- 1 cauliflower (broken into florets)
- 1 tsp. turmeric
- 1 large potato (peeled and diced)
- 4 ¼ cups hot Vegetable Stock (see recipe in Vegan Basics)
- fresh parsley or cilantro for garnish

Directions:

First, roast the garlic. This can be done ahead of time. I like to roast a couple of bulbs at once and use them in different recipes over the course of a few days.

Preheat the oven to 400°F (200°C)

Cut the top off the head of the garlic so that you can just see the tops of the cloves. Sit the garlic on a large square of aluminum foil (shiny side up) and drizzle a small amount of the olive oil over it.

Pull up the edges of the foil into a baggy parcel and put the garlic in the pre-heated oven for 40 minutes.

Remove and allow to cool a little before handling for the soup.

Make the Soup:

Pour the rest of the oil into a wide saucepan and fry the onion gently for 10 minutes or so until softened but not browning.

Add the cauliflower florets and stir in with the onion.

Add the turmeric and keep stirring, then stir in the potato.

Cover and cook over low to medium heat for about 10 minutes.

Squeeze in the baked garlic cloves (just squish the head straight into the saucepan), and add the stock/broth.

Bring to a boil, lower the heat to a simmer, then cover and cook for a further 15 minutes or so.

Purée in a food processor or blender, or, if you like a soup with more texture, use the immersion blender for a few minutes.

Add freshly chopped parsley or coriander/cilantro to serve.

> *Here's an idea to use some extra bulbs of roasted garlic: Add one to a batch of vegan mashed potatoes for a taste sensation! Just replace dairy butter and milk with Vegan Butter and any plant-based milk. Kind comfort food!*

Snacks and Appetizers

1. Spiced Roasted Garbanzo Beans

These can be eaten like a snack or used instead of croutons on a salad.

Ingredients

- 1 15 oz. can garbanzo beans (chickpeas), rinsed and drained (or 1½ cups cooked garbanzo beans)
- ½ Tbsp. organic garlic powder
- ½ Tbsp. organic onion powder
- ⅛ tsp. ground turmeric (more or less, to taste)
- dash ground black pepper
- Sprinkle of paprika

Directions:

Preheat the oven to 400°F (200°C). Line a rimmed baking sheet.

Place the garbanzo beans in a bowl, sprinkle about 2/3 of the spices over them, then bake for 15 minutes.

Remove the baking sheet from the oven and shake the beans to turn them over and sprinkle the remaining spices. Bake for another 15 minutes. Serve.

Another option for spices: Taco seasoning is also great on garbanzo beans. Toss the beans in a bowl with a splash of olive oil and the seasonings to spread evenly. Roast for 10 to 15 minutes, shake to turn them over and roast another 10 to 15 minutes.

To make your own taco seasoning so you can control the salt:

Ingredients:

- 1 Tbsp. chili powder
- ¼ tsp. garlic powder
- ¼ tsp. onion powder
- ¼ tsp. red pepper flakes
- ¼ tsp. oregano
- ½ tsp. paprika
- 1 ½ tsp. ground cumin
- 1 tsp. sea salt
- 1 tsp. black pepper

Directions:

Mix in a small bowl, then store in an airtight container.

2. Broccoli and Spinach Patties

Ingredients:

- 1 ½ cups spinach, finely chopped
- ½ cup broccoli florets, chopped
- ¼ cup grated carrot
- 1 tsp. ginger, grated
- 2 green chilis, chopped
- ½ cup garbanzo flour
- ½ tsp. red chili powder
- ½ tsp. garam masala powder
- ½ tsp. chat masala
- 1 ½ tsp. lemon juice
- Salt, to taste
- ½ cup gluten-free oats

Directions:

Heat a safe non-stick skillet (or preferably cast iron) over medium heat.

In a bowl, add all the ingredients, knead, and tightly squeeze until you get a nice ball of dough.

Form the patties to desired shape.

Once the pan is hot, place the patties in the skillet a few at a time and cook them on medium heat. When they become golden brown on one side, flip and cook on the other side.

It is very important to cook them over medium heat so they become crispy on the outside, but also cooked on the inside. Do not cook them in a hurry.

Repeat the process for the remaining dough.

Serve hot and enjoy.

&

3. Beet Hummus

Beets are good on so many levels, try to incorporate them often. This is a particularly tasty way!

Ingredients:

- 1 (15-oz) can garbanzo beans
- 1 garlic clove
- 1 medium cooked beet, peeled and quartered
- 1-2 Tbsp. tahini
- 1 lemon, juice and zest
- salt, pepper (to taste)
- vegetables or grain-free crackers (for dipping)

Directions:

Drain garbanzo beans, reserving the liquid. Set aside.

In a food processor, pulse the garlic clove until it is minced.

Add the roasted or steamed beet and pulse until finely chopped.

Scrape down the sides of the food processor, then add the garbanzo beans, tahini, lemon juice, and lemon zest.

Puree until smooth, adding garbanzo-bean liquid 1 tablespoon at a time, as needed, to achieve a smooth and creamy consistency.

Season with salt and pepper.

To cook beets, you can roast, steam, or boil:

Roasted Beets: Preheat the oven to 400°F (200°C) and line a rimmed baking sheet with parchment paper. Remove the greens but save them. They are very nutritious. Rinse the beets, peel them, and cut into wedges. Bake for 25-30 minutes, or until fork tender.

I normally boil the beets and cook several of them at a time so I can pickle some. Here is the recipe for pickled beets:

4. **Quick Pickled Spicy Beets**

Ingredients:

- 8 medium fresh beets
- 1 cup vinegar
- ½ cup sugar
- 1 ½ tsp. whole cloves

- 1 ½ tsp. whole allspice
- ½ tsp. salt

Directions:

Clean and boil the beets. Scrub them and trim the tops down to 1 inch. (Again - don't toss the greens!)

Place the beets in a large pot and add water to cover. Bring the mixture to a boil, then reduce heat and simmer, covered, 25-30 minutes or until tender.

Remove the beets from water and let cool. One they are cool to the touch, peel and slice them, set aside. You can use a small bowl, or if you're planning on using them as a garnish, put them in a jar.

Mix the Brine:

In a small saucepan, combine the vinegar, sugar, cloves, allspice, and salt. Bring to a boil for 5 minutes. Pour the mixture over the beets in the jar or bowl.

Refrigerate at least 1 hour. Drain before serving.

I sometimes use these as a side dish for a meal, especially the Lentil Shepherd's Pie – or they are a nutritious snack.

The beets last at least a month in the fridge.

When the beets are all gone, I use the brine in a veggie smoothie.

International Flavors

1. Falafel

There are literally hundreds of recipes for falafel because it is a staple in many cultures, but I have used this one many times, and love it.

This first recipe is just for the falafel – but you may want to serve it with tzatziki – check the recipe to make sure you have the ingredients.

To prep for this recipe, you will need to soak the garbanzo beans overnight if you're going to cook from dried. Be sure there's plenty of water covering them – at least 2 inches above the top.

Ingredients:

- 1 cup cooked garbanzo beans (chickpeas), or 1 15 oz. can
- 1 cup roughly chopped onion
- 2 Tbsp. finely chopped fresh parsley
- 2 Tbsp. finely chopped fresh cilantro
- 1 tsp. salt
- ½ -1 tsp. hot chili peppers
- 4 cloves garlic
- 1 tsp. cumin
- 1 tsp. baking powder
- 4-6 Tbsp. almond or rice flour (you can use regular flour if you are not sensitive to wheat, but it can cause inflammation, so I do not recommend it)

- Avocado oil for frying

Directions:

Place the drained garbanzo beans and the onions in the bowl of a food processor.

Add the parsley, cilantro, salt, hot pepper, garlic, and cumin.

Process until blended but not like cake batter. You still want some texture.

Sprinkle the baking powder and 4 tablespoons of whatever flour you're using, and pulse. The idea is to add enough flour so that the dough forms a small ball and does not stick to your hands.

Put it into a bowl with a cover and refrigerate for 4 hours or more.

When you're ready to cook, form the dough into balls about the size of walnuts.

Heat the oil to 375°F in a wok or deep frying pan. Start with just one ball and test whether they will hold up. If it falls apart, add flour a little at a time.

Fry just a few balls at once until they're golden brown, a few minutes on each side.

Drain on paper towels.

Serve with chopped tomato, green onions, or whatever else you like to garnish.

Normally, falafel is served with a cucumber (tzatziki) sauce or tahini sauce and often with pita bread.

In this brain-healthy lifestyle, I recommend staying away from the flour products, but I've provided you with recipes for a couple of grain-free bread substitutes (see in Vegan Basics) so you could serve either of them with the falafel.

This recipe freezes very well, so make a batch and freeze some for later. Cook once, eat twice!

2. Vegan Tzatziki Sauce

This is a great tzatziki sauce. It's easy and delicious. Traditionally, this sauce uses Greek yogurt, but we're not going to go that way. First, we don't do dairy (right?), and second, Greek yogurt production results in a toxic waste substance (acid whey) that is so environmentally damaging, it is illegal to dump it into waterways.

I use coconut milk yogurt and make my own because I live in Ecuador. (The recipe is included in the Vegan Basics section of the recipes). But if you can get your hands on a plain coconut or other plant-based thick yogurt, store-bought is just fine. Just buy the thickest you can. If the yogurt is thin, pour it over a couple of layers of cheesecloth spread over a mesh strainer set atop a bowl or large measuring cup and strain several hours or overnight until a good solid yogurt remains on top.

Ingredients:

- 1 medium, or ½ large cucumber. Don't peel it – grate it to get about 1 cup of cucumber.
- 1½ cups coconut milk or other thick plant-based yogurt
- 3 cloves minced garlic
- 2 Tbsp. dried dill (If you have fresh, that's even better, in which case you want about ¼ cup, chopped.)
- 1½ Tbsp. lemon juice
- A pinch of sea salt and black pepper (to taste)

Directions:

Finely grate the cucumber and extract the water by squeezing through a nut bag or cheesecloth. You want about ¼ cup of cucumber for the sauce.

Put the yogurt, strained cucumber, and remaining ingredients into a bowl and mix well.

Taste test – add more of whatever you think it needs.

Use immediately or store in the fridge. It lasts about 5 days, although I'm guessing you'll gobble it up before then!

☙

3. Zucchini Fritters

I like serving these with the tzatziki sauce in the recipe above, so if you're making a batch of that, maybe plan this for the next day after falafel!

Have three or four clean linen kitchen towels handy to gently wring the water out of the grated vegetables. It's better to use a box grater than a food processor for this recipe.

Ingredients:

- 2 Tbsp. flax meal
- ½ cup room temperature water
- 2 large zucchini (about 4 cups shredded/pre-squeezed)
- ½ cup shredded potato
- ½ cup shredded carrot
- ½ cup shredded onion
- ⅓ cup chopped herb mixture – parsley and/or mint and/or thyme
- 1 Tbsp. lemon zest
- ½ cup finely ground oats or, if you're concerned about inflammation, you can finely crush walnuts in a spice or coffee mill
- ½ cup almond flour
- 1 tsp. aluminum free baking powder
- 1 tsp. salt (plus 2 tsp. to pull moisture out of zucchini)
- ½ tsp. freshly ground black pepper
- ¼ tsp. ground nutmeg
- approx. ½ cup avocado oil (or light olive oil) for frying

Instructions

Shred zucchini into colander and sprinkle with about 2 teaspoons of salt to draw out the moisture. Drain it over the sink for 20 minutes or so.

Mix flax meal and water until completely combined. Set aside for 10 minutes to thicken.

Shred onions, carrots, and potatoes. Squeeze out liquid from onions and potatoes by ringing them in a clean kitchen/tea towel. Set aside.

Chop herbs, measure out ground walnuts or oats and spices.

Mix chopped herbs, ground walnuts or oats, lemon zest, and spices in a large bowl.

When flax meal is ready, mix into the bowl with herbs/crumbs/spices and baking powder until completely combined.

Very lightly rinse shredded zucchini (to get rid of the salt) and ring out any liquid in a kitchen/tea towel.

Add all shredded veggies to the bowl with flax mixture and stir to combine completely.

Add the almond flour and, working with your hands, combine everything.

Set aside to rest for at least 10 minutes on the counter.

Add 3 tablespoons oil to shallow frying pan and bring to medium heat.

When ready to fry, scoop up about 1/3 cup of squash mixture and roll into a ball in your hands. Add ball to hot pan and gently pat into a patty.

Leave room between patties so you can easily flip them. Be careful not to scorch the oil. Fry for about 2 or 3 minutes on each side to a crispy golden brown.

Add more oil to the pan between batches.

Drain on paper towels and serve hot.

&

4. Baba Ghanoush

This is a yummy dip filled with the goodness of sesame seeds, eggplant, garlic, and lemon. It is traditionally served with pita bread, but we're serving it with celery, carrot, and pepper sticks, or with the Yucca (or Cassava) Flour Tortillas (See Vegan Basics).

Ingredients:

- 2 medium eggplants
- 2 cloves garlic, crushed
- 1 lemon, juiced
- 4 Tbsp. tahini
- 2 Tbsp. olive oil
- ½ tsp. ground cumin
- smoked paprika
- 1 Tbsp. parsley, chopped

Directions:

Preheat the oven to 450°F (230°C). Line a large baking tray with baking paper.

Halve the eggplants lengthwise and brush the cut sides lightly with olive oil. Place them in the prepared tray with the halved sides down, roasting them for 35-40 minutes until the flesh is very tender.

Once the eggplants are cooked, set them aside to cool, then scoop out the flesh with a spoon, discarding the skin.

Place the flesh on a sieve and leave for a bit (the longer, the better) to allow all the excess liquid to drain away.

Place the flesh in a bowl, add the garlic, lemon juice, tahini, olive oil, and cumin. Mash everything with a fork and continue stirring and mashing until the mixture is creamy. Season to taste with salt.

Transfer to a serving bowl and sprinkle with smoked paprika and chopped parsley to garnish.

5. **Plantain Mangu** (Dominican Republic)

Ingredients:

- 5 green bananas (plantains verde) cut in 1-inch slices
- 3 Tbsp. Vegan Butter (in Vegan Basics)
- water to boil the plantains
- salt to taste
- 3 green onions
- olive oil to add to mash

Directions:

Boil the peeled and cut plantains in salted water until they are soft.

Strain the plantains, then mash while they are hot, adding the olive oil and a little water or plant milk to result in a puree similar to mashed potatoes.

Serve warm with green onions sprinkled on top. This is delicious in the Yucca Flour Tortillas (see Vegan Basics) with spicy salsa and some black beans, or you can dip veggie sticks or grain-free crackers and use it like an appetizer.

6. **Boronía (Mashed Plantain and Eggplant)** (Colombia)

This is a traditional dish from the Atlantic coast of Colombia. It is served as a side dish but can also be an appetizer served with chips.

Ingredients:

- 3 large ripe plantains, peeled and diced

- 1 large eggplant, peeled and diced
- 2 Tbsp. olive oil
- Salt
- Fresh ground pepper

For the Tomato Mixture to go on top of plantain mixture:
- 1 cup chopped tomato
- 2 large garlic cloves
- 3 scallions, chopped
- ½ Tbsp. olive or avocado oil
- 3 Tbsp. grated Vegan Mozzarella (in Vegan Basics)

Directions:

Preheat oven to 350°F (175°C).

Place the eggplant and plantains in a baking dish and drizzle with 2 table-spoons olive oil. Bake for 25 minutes.

While that's cooking, heat the oil in a safe non-stick pan over medium heat. Add the tomato, onion, garlic, salt, and pepper and cook, stirring occasionally for 10 minutes.

Set aside, keeping the mixture warm.

Process the baked eggplant and plantains in a food processor just until they are combined. Do not over process – you don't want them to be like a puree.

Transfer the eggplant and plantain mixture to a serving bowl. Cover with the tomato mixture and mozzarella cheese and mix well. Serve hot.

Fermented Foods

1. Cabbage Juice

Ingredients:

- 3 cups coarsely chopped organic red cabbage
- ¾ cup filtered water
- 1 tsp. sea salt

Directions:

Fill the blender with the chopped cabbage, salt, and water. Blend gently on a low speed so that you get small pieces, not a puree. Pour the blended mixture in a jar that allows room for expansion. Cover the jar and let the mixture sit for three days at room temperature.

After three days, strain the mixture to separate the juice and pulp. Put the fermented juice in the refrigerator and aim for drinking ½ cup per day diluted with equal parts of water.

(Recipe adapted from HealthyandNaturalWorld.com)

2. Sauerkraut

I only make sauerkraut in jars rather than in big crocks – it's easier to monitor. This recipe makes one 1-quart jar.

Ingredients:

- 1 medium head green cabbage
- Non-iodized salt (pure sea salt or pink salt, which is what I use)

Directions:

Take the outer leaves off the cabbage and save one or two of the cleanest good-sized ones because you'll be using that to cover the kraut in the jar.

Quarter the cabbage and take out the core.

Grate or slice the cabbage very finely. You want to make lots of surface area for the salt to get into the cabbage. You can use a food processor, but I cut it by hand. No chunks!

Weigh the cabbage – 1.75 pounds, or about 800 grams, is perfect for a 1-quart jar.

Add 16 grams of salt* (.56 ounces)

> *It's important to ensure you have the right proportion of salt. The ratio is 50 to 1 – so 50 grams of cabbage to 1 gram of salt. 16 grams of salt is about 1 tablespoon of salt. But because different salts can have different densities, it is best to go by weight.*

Mix it together well in a mixing bowl, massaging the salt into the cabbage. I let it sit for 10 or 15 minutes, then continue massaging in the salt and squishing the cabbage to get lots of brine. You should have a little puddle in the bottom of the bowl when you tilt it to the side.

Stuff the whole mixture into the jar, packing tightly (but not too tightly). Continue pressing the cabbage to get as much brine going as possible. The cabbage and brine should get to about 1 ½ inches from the top so you have room for a weight. Be sure to put any of the brine from the bowl into the jar as well.

Most important: Make sure the brine completely covers the cabbage all the time.

Put the clean cabbage leaf on top of the mixture and press down. Be sure to have the brine cover the kraut, and you'll want to make sure all the time it's fermenting that the cabbage stays below the brine. Use a weight to keep the cabbage below the brine (you can buy commercial fermenting weights or a sterile rock or even use a small freezer bag filled with salt water – 1 tablespoon salt to 2 cups of water). Screw the lid on the top but leave it a bit loose so the gases can escape.

Now ferment. Put the jar in a shallow bowl to catch the brine that will probably leak out during the first week. Keep the jar out of direct sunlight and excess heat.

In the first few days you'll see little bubbles forming and likely some liquid will escape from the loose lid. Every day, open the lid to let the gases escape but make sure the brine still covers the cabbage. After a few days it won't bubble anymore. Just leave it closed (lid not tight because you still want the gasses to escape). Let it sit for two to four weeks – just watch that the brine covers the cabbage.

This is a very rudimentary recipe, but the one I use all the time. If you're nervous or have never done anything like this before, go online. There are literally dozens of videos and recipes with photos.

(Recipe adapted from family tradition)

3. Simple Cabbage Kimchi

I love kimchi because I like spicy foods. It is also easy and is ready in just a couple of days, although it does take some time to make. You'll want to use gloves to mix this because of the red pepper.

Ingredients:

- 1 head Napa cabbage (2 pounds or so)
- ¼ cup iodine-free sea salt or pink salt
- Filtered water
- 1 Tbsp. grated garlic
- 1 Tbsp. grated peeled fresh ginger
- 1 tsp. sugar

- 3 Tbsp. water
- 1 to 5 Tbsp. Korean red pepper flakes (gochugaru) (I only use 1 Tbsp. if I can get it – it's hot. If you can't get this, just use regular red (chili) pepper flakes.)
- 8 oz. daikon or Korean radish, peeled and cut into matchsticks. I can't get this here in Ecuador all the time, so I normally just use regular red radishes. They work very well. If you use them, just be sure they are solid.
- 4 medium scallions, trimmed and cut into 1-inch pieces

Directions:

Cut the cabbage lengthwise through the stem into quarters. Cut the cores from each piece. Cut each quarter into strips.

Place the cabbage in a large bowl and sprinkle with the salt. Massage the salt into the cabbage until it starts to soften a bit. Add enough water to cover the cabbage. Put a plate on top of the cabbage and weigh it down with something heavy and let it stand for an hour or two.

Rinse the cabbage under cold water 3 times. You want to get all the salt and brine off the mixture. Set aside to drain in a colander for 15 to 20 minutes.

While that's draining, make the spice paste. Add the garlic, ginger, sugar, and water and stir into a smooth paste in a large bowl. Stir in the red pepper. Set this aside until the cabbage is completely drained.

Gently squeeze any remaining water from the cabbage and add it to the spice paste. Add the radish and scallions.

With gloved hands, gently work the paste into the vegetables until they are thoroughly coated.

Pack the kimchi into a 1-quart jar. Press down on the kimchi until the brine (the liquid that comes out) rises to cover the vegetables, leaving at least 1 inch of space at the top. Seal the jar.

Let it ferment for 1 to 5 days. Place a shallow bowl under the jar to catch any overflow. Like the sauerkraut, you want to keep the kimchi out of direct sunlight, at cool room temperature. Let it sit for 1 to 5 days. You will also see bubbles – open the jar and let the gases escape – but you don't need weights because you are going to keep pressing down on the veggies with a spoon to make sure they stay submerged.

You can taste the kimchi every day and stop the fermentation whenever you feel it is the right taste for you. Just be sure to use a clean fork or spoon every time you try it and be sure to submerge the vegetables each time.

Move the jar to the refrigerator to stop the fermentation. Let it sit for another week in the fridge for best taste, although you can eat it right away.

There are also dozens of recipes for kimchi online – and plenty of videos to help in case you're a visual learner.

Holiday Yummies

The memories we share thanks to holidays are usually centered around food. Now that you're enjoying this healthy lifestyle, you may find it a bit of a challenge to share meals with meat-eating friends and family members who don't understand your choices.

But this is an incredible opportunity to make delicious meals that can demonstrate that, not only are you not giving up anything, you are enjoying delicious foods AND looking after your health and your brain.

So here are some beautiful and tasty vegan recipes for Thanksgiving, Christmas, and Hanukkah.

Christmas and/or Thanksgiving

1. **Beet Hummus** (#3 in Snacks and Appetizers) is colorful and delicious. Add some carrots, celery, and green pepper spears on the serving plate and you have the perfect Christmas appetizer.

2. **Christmas Vegetables**

Ingredients:

- 4 Tbsp. extra virgin olive oil
- ½ pound mixed colored carrots, peeled and chopped
- ½ pound potatoes, peeled and chopped
- ½ pound sweet potatoes, peeled and chopped
- ½ pound parsnips peeled and chopped
- 2 red onions roughly chopped
- 5 garlic cloves, peeled
- 4 beets, washed and halved
- 1 orange, cut into thin slices
- 1 Tbsp. dried rosemary
- 1 Tbsp. dried thyme

- Pink or sea salt and pepper to taste
- 1 handful of fresh thyme, chopped (for serving)

Directions:

Preheat the oven to 400ºF (200ºC)

Add the oil to the bottom of a large roasting tray and place in the oven for 5 minutes.

Once the oil is warm, add the vegetables, dried herbs, whole garlic cloves and salt and pepper.

Toss the vegetables until they are well coated and bake for 30 to 35 minutes or until slightly crispy. Halfway through baking, gently toss the vegetables and add a sparse layer of orange slices evenly on top.

Once the vegetables are cooked, garnish with fresh thyme and salt.

Serve hot.

3. Vegan Stuffing Balls

Ingredients:

- 2 onions, finely diced
- ½ cup vegetable broth
- 14 oz. gluten free breadcrumbs*
- 2 cups chestnut or cremini mushrooms, sliced
- 2 oz. Vegan Butter (see in Vegan Basics)
- 1 Tbsp. extra virgin olive oil
- 1 tsp. dried thyme
- 1 tsp. dried basil
- 1 tsp. dried rosemary
- 1 tsp. dried marjoram

- 1 tsp. sage
- Pink or sea salt and pepper to taste

Directions:

Preheat the oven to 350ºF (175ºC).

Heat the oil and onions in a pan on medium heat and cook for 5 minutes, stirring constantly.

Add a generous pinch of salt and pepper and the sliced mushrooms to the pan. Cook for 10 minutes, or until they are brown and most of the moisture has evaporated.

Transfer the onions and mushrooms to a large mixing bowl and add the breadcrumbs.

Add all of the remaining ingredients and stir thoroughly.

Form the stuffing mixture into balls and place them on a lightly greased rimmed baking sheet.

Cover with another of the same kind of baking sheet (to avoid use of aluminum foil) and bake for 20 minutes.

Allow to cool slightly before serving.

> **Grain warning: As you know we try to avoid grains on this plan, but sometimes, for special occasions, it's okay to indulge as long as you don't have serious inflammation issues.*

4. Lentil "Meatless" Loaf

Ingredients:

- 2 ¼ cups cooked lentils (or two cans of prepared lentils) drained
- 1 cup walnuts, finely chopped
- 2 tsp. extra-virgin olive oil
- 2 cups finely chopped yellow onion
- 4 cloves garlic, minced
- 1 cup finely chopped celery
- 1 cup grated carrot
- 1 cup cremini mushrooms, roughly chopped (see Note re: cleaning mushrooms)
- 1 tsp. rubbed thyme
- 1 tsp. dried oregano
- 1 tsp. pink salt (more or less, to taste)
- ¼ tsp. freshly ground black pepper (more or less, to taste)
- 3 Tbsp. ground flax
- ½ cup oat flour
- ¼ tsp. red pepper flakes (optional)

Directions:

Preheat the oven to 325°F (160°C).

Spread the chopped walnuts onto a baking sheet. Toast the nuts for 8 to 12 minutes until fragrant and slightly golden. Set aside to cool.

Grease a 9x5-inch loaf pan, and then line it with a piece of parchment paper or a silicon mat cut to fit the length of the pan.

After draining the lentils, put 1½ cups of them in the food processor and grind them into a paste. Leave the remaining ½ cup of lentils whole.

Put all of the lentils into a large bowl.

Increase the oven to 350°F (180°C).

Heat the oil in a large skillet on medium heat.

Once the oil is shimmering, stir in the onion and garlic and a dash of salt.

Cook, stirring frequently, for 4 to 5 minutes until the onion softens.

Stir in the celery and carrot and continue cooking until they are also slightly soft.

Stir in the mushrooms, thyme, oregano, 1/2 tsp. salt, and black pepper. Cook for a couple minutes longer.

Into the bowl with the lentils, stir in the walnuts, ground flax, oat flour, and mix until combined.

Stir in all of the veggie mixture until combined.

Add the red pepper flakes, if using.

Taste and add more salt and/or pepper if desired.

If the mixture seems dry, add a tablespoon or two of water and mix again.

Press all of the lentil loaf mixture into the prepared loaf pan. Pack it down firmly to ensure it holds together.

Bake the lentil loaf, uncovered, for 50 to 60 minutes until the edges start to darken and the loaf is semi-firm to the touch.

Once done, place the loaf pan directly onto a cooling rack for 15 minutes.

After the loaf has cooled for 15 minutes, put an appropriately shaped plate on top of the loaf pan and invert the pan to allow the loaf to slide out onto the plate.

Cool on the rack for at least another 15 minutes if you can wait! Otherwise it will crumble a bit.

Serve with the following amazingly delicious mushroom gravy (recipe #5).

The vegan stuffing balls (recipe #3 above) along with vegan mashed potatoes make excellent traditional accompaniments for a vegan Christmas feast featuring this loaf.

Note: For cleaning mushrooms, use a damp paper towel or a soft brush to clean each mushroom individually. You can also lightly rinse the mushrooms with water, but don't soak them. Pat dry when done.

5. Vegan Mushroom Gravy

Ingredients:

- 3 Tbsp. vegan butter (See Vegan Basics)
- 1 cup diced red onion
- 1 lb cremini mushrooms, sliced
- 4 medium garlic cloves, minced
- ¼ tsp. dried thyme
- 1 Tbsp. vegan Worcestershire
- 3 Tbsp. non-GMO cornstarch or tapioca flour to thicken the gravy
- 3 cups Vegetable Broth (See Vegan Basics)
- 1 Tbsp. chives

Directions:

Melt the butter in a large sauté pan over medium heat.

Add the sliced mushrooms and diced onions to the pan and sauté for 10 minutes.

The onions may get a little brown and stick to the pan, but just use a wooden spatula and scrape any brown bits off the bottom of the pan.

Add the minced garlic, 1/4 tsp dried thyme, 1 tbsp vegan Worcestershire sauce, and 1 tbsp low-sodium tamari to the pan. Stir and let it cook for 1 minute.

Add 3 tbsp cornstarch or flour and stir to coat the mushrooms. Let it cook for 1 minute, stirring occasionally.

Add 3 cups of vegetable broth and stir it all together until you don't see any clumps of flour.

Bring the gravy to a low simmer (look for small bubbles) and then reduce the heat to medium-low. Let it cook for 10 minutes while the gravy continues to thicken.

Serve the gravy over the Lentil "Meatless" Loaf, in recipe 4 above, along with mashed potatoes and a colorful vegetable like broccoli and you have a delicious holiday meal.

*Note: You can store the leftovers in an airtight container in the fridge for 4-5 days or freeze it for several months. It tends to thicken up when it's stored in the fridge and freezer, so you may need to add 1-2 tbsp of vegetable broth or water to thin the gravy when you reheat it.

Hanukkah

6. Challah made with Aquafaba

While there is a bit of sugar and gluten-free flour, Challah is almost essential at this time of year, and it just doesn't work well without flour. So as long as you're not wheat sensitive, and you are careful to eat plenty of other things to counteract any potential for inflammation, it's fine to make an exception.

This is a lot of work, but it will be worth it to have this special treat.

Ingredients:

- 1 Tbsp. active dry yeast
- 1 cup water, divided
- ¼ cup aquafaba (liquid from a can of garbanzo beans)

- 6 tsp. sugar, divided
- ¾ tsp. kosher salt, plus more for sprinkling
- ¼ cup hemp or avocado oil, divided
- 3 ½ cups gluten-free flour (this is one of the few times I use flour)
- 2 Tbsp. non-dairy milk
- 1 Tbsp. maple syrup

Directions:

In a small bowl, place ¼ cup warm tap water, and stir in 1 ½ teaspoon of sugar.

Sprinkle the yeast over the top and allow to sit for about 5-10 minutes. The yeast will become cloudy and dissolve.

In the bowl of your stand mixer, add ¾ cup water, ¼ cup aquafaba, 2 tablespoons oil, ¾ teaspoon salt, and the remaining sugar. Whisk well to combine.

Add the yeast.

Attach the dough hook to your stand mixer and put the bowl in place. Turn on at a low speed and start to add the flour, a little at a time, until it is all incorporated. The dough should be smooth and not tacky. You can also do this step by hand, but it's a lot more work.

Form the dough into a ball and rub it all over with about a tablespoon of oil. Place it back into the bowl, cover with a clean cloth, and allow to rise in a warm spot for about 90 minutes.

Pull the dough out of the bowl and punch it down. Divide it into 6 equal balls. Roll each ball out to a rope about 12 inches long. Mush three strands together at the top, then braid them, mushing them together at the end as well. Place on a parchment-lined cookie sheet, then repeat with the other loaf.

In a small bowl, mix together the vegan milk and the maple syrup, then brush it all over the tops of both loaves. Sprinkle with a little kosher salt, or poppyseeds or sesame seeds.

Bake in a preheated 350°F (175°C) oven for about 30-40 minutes, until the tops are golden. Remove from oven and allow to cool enough to slice. Best eaten warm.

Passover

7. Matzo-Ball Soup

Ingredients:

For the Vegetable Soup:

- 2 Tbsp. olive oil
- 1 large onion, finely chopped
- 3 celery stalks, diced
- 4 cups Vegetable Broth (See Vegan Basics)
- 6 medium potatoes, peeled and finely diced
- 6-8 medium carrots, sliced
- Handful of celery leaves
- 1 Tbsp. all-purpose seasoning
- ¼ cup chopped fresh dill, or to taste
- Salt and freshly ground black pepper, to taste

For the Matzo Balls:

- 1 cup quinoa flakes
- 2 cups boiling water
- 1 cup matzo meal or for gluten free, substitute 1¼ cups quinoa flakes
- ¼ cup avocado oil
- ¼ tsp. salt
- Freshly cracked black pepper
- Pinch of onion and/or garlic powder, optional

Directions:

For the Vegetable Soup:

Heat olive oil in a large soup pot. Add the onion and celery and sauté over medium heat until golden.

Add the broth, potato, carrots, celery leaves, seasoning blend, and 2 cups water.

Bring to a rapid simmer, then cover and simmer gently for 15 to 20 minutes, until the vegetables are tender.

Stir in the dill, then season with salt and pepper.

*See Notes for advance preparation.

Just before serving, bring to a simmer. Adjust consistency with more water if needed, and taste to adjust seasonings. Add warmed matzo balls to individual servings.

For the Matzo Balls:

In a large mixing bowl, cover quinoa flakes with the water. Let stand for 2-3 minutes.

Stir in the matzo meal along with the oil and mix until well blended. Cover the bowl and refrigerate for at least 15 minutes.

Just before baking, preheat the oven to 275°F (135°C).

Roll the matzo meal mixture into approximately 1-inch balls; don't pack them too firmly.

Arrange on a parchment-lined baking sheet.

Bake for 20-25 minutes, carefully turning them after 10 minutes, until firm to the touch; don't let them brown.

Distribute them among the soup bowls, allowing three or four matzo balls per serving.

*See Notes if you make these in advance.

Notes:

This soup is especially good if you allow it to sit for an hour or so to allow the flavors to meld. It can also be made the day before serving, then heated to simmering before adding the matzo balls.

If you are making the matzo balls ahead of time, let them cool completely. Cover until needed and heat up briefly in a medium oven before serving.

Natural Cleaning Products

1. **Laundry Detergent** (Recipe thanks to Food Revolution)

This recipe includes essential oils for scent, but if you prefer unscented laundry detergent, then leave them out.

Ingredients:

- 2 cups grated bar soap (try for something all-natural like shea butter soap base, available online at places like Bulk Apothecary)
- 4 cups washing soda (aka soda ash) (available at Amazon and in some grocery stores or in hardware stores)
- 4 cups borax (available in most grocery stores)
- Optional: ¼ tsp. or 50 drops lemon essential oil
- Optional: ¼ tsp. or 50 drops lavender essential oil

Directions:

In a large bowl, mix the grated soap, washing soda, and borax.

If you are using the oils, slowly add them in as you are mixing the other ingredients.

Pour the mixture into a large mason jar. It's always best to store things in glass if possible.

Use ¼ to ½ cup per load of laundry.

&

2. All-Purpose Spray Cleaner 1

Fill a big jar with lemon and/or lime rinds.

Top it up with vinegar. Let it ferment for three weeks, then strain the liquid into a container.

It is an amazing all-purpose cleaner and leaves your house smelling like a lemon grove!

&

3. All-Purpose Spray Cleaner 2

Ingredients:

- ½ tsp. washing soda (aka soda ash) (available at Amazon and in some grocery stores or in hardware stores)
- ½ cup liquid soap (like castile)
- 2 cups very hot tap water
- *Optional: 50 drops of lemon essential oil

Directions:

Combine all the ingredients in a spray bottle and shake until the washing soda has dissolved.

For tough dirt, leave the cleaner on the sprayed surface for a few minutes before wiping it off.

&

4. Toilet Bowl Cleaner

Dump equal parts (at least ½ cup) vinegar and baking soda into the toilet. Let it foam and sit a few minutes, then scrub.

For extra-tough cleaning jobs – scrub with the brush as you flush and the water empties out. Fill the bowl with white vinegar and allow to sit overnight. Scrub in the morning with brush. You can add a little extra baking soda at the same time if it's still stained.

References

Chapter 1

1   https://www.ahnphealth.com/dr-bredesen.html

2   https://www.alzforum.org/early-onset-familial-ad/diagnosisgenetics/genetic-testing-and-counseling-early-onset-familial

3   https://alz-journals.onlinelibrary.wiley.com/doi/full/10.1002/alz.12001

4   https://www.mayoclinic.org/diseases-conditions/vascular-dementia/symptoms-causes/syc-20378793

5   https://www.mayoclinic.org/diseases-conditions/lewy-body-dementia/symptoms-causes/syc-20352025

6   https://www.cbsnews.com/news/kris-kristofferson-misdiagnosed-alzheimers-has-lyme-disease/

7   https://www.bbc.com/news/health-26480756

8   https://www.alzheimers.net/12-3-14-blood-test-detects-alzheimers-early/

9   https://www.j-alz.com/content/study-reveals-association-between-physical-function-and-neurological-disease

10   https://www.sciencedaily.com/releases/2019/08/190801162144.htm

11   https://www.bmc.org/news/press-releases/2019/03/21/new-study-finds-test-protein-levels-eye-potential-predictor-future

12   https://medicalxpress.com/news/2020-07-blood-alzheimer-markers-tau-closer.html

13   https://www.aao.org/eye-health/news/retina-scan-early-warning-of-alzheimers-disease

14   https://www.sciencedaily.com/releases/2019/05/190523202607.htm

Chapter 2

1   https://www.brucelipton.com/what-epigenetics

Chapter 3

1   https://www.theguardian.com/science/2016/aug/25/gut-reaction-surprising-power-of-microbes
2   https://www.huffpost.com/entry/leaky-gut-syndrome-what-y_b_8632880
3   https://www.medicalnewstoday.com/articles/220302#-human-parasites-
4   https://www.ncbi.nlm.nih.gov/pmc/articles/PMC6214864/
5   https://www.ncbi.nlm.nih.gov/pmc/articles/PMC4141874/
6   https://www.drperlmutter.com/wp-content/uploads/2017/12/Midlife-systemic-inflammatory-markers-are-associated-with-late-life-brain-volume.pdf
7   https://www.healthline.com/nutrition/sugar-and-inflammation#section1
8   https://www.drperlmutter.com/wp-content/uploads/2017/12/Midlife-systemic-inflammatory-markers-are-associated-with-late-life-brain-volume.pdf
9   https://holisticprimarycare.net/topics/environomics/glyphosate-a-root-cause-of-chronic-inflammation/
10   https://www.ncbi.nlm.nih.gov/pmc/articles/PMC5725362/
11   https://www.newscientist.com/article/2191814-we-may-finally-know-what-causes-alzheimers-and-how-to-stop-it/
12   https://www.healthline.com/health-news/are-alzheimers-and-gum-disease-connected
13   https://www.bcm.edu/news/fungi-cause-brain-infection-in-mice
14   https://pubmed.ncbi.nlm.nih.gov/12480795/

Chapter 4

1   https://www.mayoclinic.org/diseases-conditions/alzheimers-disease/symptoms-causes/syc-20350447
2   https://www.ncbi.nlm.nih.gov/pmc/articles/PMC4722942/
3   https://www.cell.com/neuron/fulltext/S0896-6273(17)30791-2
4   https://www.sciencedirect.com/science/article/abs/pii/S0006322309002261
5   https://www.neurologyadvisor.com/topics/neurodegenerative-diseases/obesity-and-alzheimer-disease-exploring-risk-modification/
6   https://jamanetwork.com/journals/jamaneurology/fullarticle/789626
7   https://n.neurology.org/content/92/6/e594

8   https://www.drperlmutter.com/study/inverse-association-between-bmi-and-prefrontal-metabolic-activity-in-healthy-adults/

9   https://www.alzheimers.net/10-07-15-midlife-weight-connected-to-alzheimers

10   https://www.ncbi.nlm.nih.gov/pmc/articles/PMC6054325/

11   https://www.diabetes.co.uk/news/2018/apr/artificial-sweeteners-linked-to-poor-metabolism-and-increased-Type 2-diabetes-risk-

12   https://healthy.shared.com/artificially-sweetened-drinks-aspartame-etc-found-to-triple-your-risk-of-stroke-dementia-according-to-studies/

13   https://www.pressdemocrat.com/article/news/sucralose-might-be-making-you-fatter-and-sicker-a-new-study-says/

14   https://nutritionstudies.org/the-cheese-trap-fighting-diabetes-with-a-dairy-free-diet/

15   https://pubmed.ncbi.nlm.nih.gov/1377788/

16   https://nutritionstudies.org/the-cheese-trap-fighting-diabetes-with-a-dairy-free-diet/

17   https://nutritionstudies.org/sugary-fruit-healthy/

18   https://www.pcrm.org/health-topics/diabetes

19   https://drjockers.com/insulin-resistance/

20   https://www.plantbasednews.org/lifestyle/

Chapter 5

1   https://pubmed.ncbi.nlm.nih.gov/18795985/

2   https://pubmed.ncbi.nlm.nih.gov/28294066/

3   https://www.medicalnewstoday.com/articles/320779

4   https://www.mayoclinic.org/diseases-conditions/insomnia/in-depth/insomnia-treatment/art-20046677

Chapter 6

1   https://sph.umd.edu/news-item/exercise-activates-memory-networks-older-adults

2   https://www.cuimc.columbia.edu/news/aerobic-exercise-improves-cognition-even-young-adults

3   https://www.eurekalert.org/pub_releases/2020-01/mc-eak123019.php

4   https://pubmed.ncbi.nlm.nih.gov/11485502/

5   https://www.ncbi.nlm.nih.gov/pmc/articles/PMC4789972/

6   https://www.nature.com/articles/s41591-018-0275-4

7 https://neurosciencenews.com/exercise-intensity-brain-15610/

8 https://www.nytimes.com/2018/09/10/well/move/using-tai-chi-to-build-strength.html

9 https://www.ncbi.nlm.nih.gov/pmc/articles/PMC5359459/

10 https://health.usnews.com/health-care/for-better/articles/how-aerobic-exercise-benefits-the-brain-especially-as-you-age

11 https://content.iospress.com/articles/brain-plasticity/bpl190093

12 https://www.bbc.com/news/health-1024034?inf_contact_key=24eefbe7215ec31f6b8b79823fcc1628

13 https://www.awakeningfromalzheimers.com/this-may-be-the-most-powerful-way-to-a-stronger-brain/

14 https://psychology-spot.com/dancing-makes-me-happy/

15 https://psychology-spot.com/dancing-makes-me-happy/

16 https://www.betterhealth.vic.gov.au/health/conditionsandtreatments/depression-and-exercise

17 http://aginginstride.enewsworks.com/en/10024/articles/1055/Is-Depression-a-Risk-Factor-for-Alzheimer's-Disease.htm

18 https://www.sbs.com.au/news/weights-may-help-stop-alzheimer-s-study

Chapter 7

1 https://www.sciencedirect.com/science/article/pii/S0269749119348511

2 https://pubmed.ncbi.nlm.nih.gov/21157018/

3 https://pubmed.ncbi.nlm.nih.gov/24577474/

4 http://www.second-opinions.co.uk/teflon_alzheimers.html#.XwtAKxOSk2x

5 https://www.ewg.org/research/canaries-kitchen#.WdTot8lrzBI

6 https://www.ncbi.nlm.nih.gov/pmc/articles/PMC2920088/

7 https://www.beingpatient.com/air-pollution-risk-of-alzheimers/

8 https://ehjournal.biomedcentral.com/articles/10.1186/s12940-020-0565-4

9 https://www.sciencemag.org/news/2017/01/brain-pollution-evidence-builds-dirty-air-causes-alzheimer-s-dementia

10 https://www.pnas.org/content/115/21/E4853

11 https://pubmed.ncbi.nlm.nih.gov/25072238/

12 https://pubmed.ncbi.nlm.nih.gov/19539684/

13 https://www.askdrray.com/toxins-in-the-bathroom/

14 https://www.fda.gov/cosmetics/potential-contaminants-cosmetics/fdas-testing-cosmetics-arsenic-cadmium-chromium-cobalt-lead-mercury-and-nickel-content#top

15 https://www.sfgate.com/health/article/What-s-in-furniture-It-s-enough-to-make-you-sick-3237613.php

16 https://www.drperlmutter.com/study/circulatory-levels-of-toxic-metals-in-patients-with-alzheimers-disease/

17 https://www.healthline.com/health/alzheimers-dementia/dementia-due-to-metabolic-causes#prevention

18 https://www.rfsafe.com/radiation-cell-phones-cause-uks-100-increase-early-dementia-starting-30/

19 https://www.ncbi.nlm.nih.gov/pmc/articles/PMC5038365/#b48-etm-0-0-3567

Chapter 8

1 https://www.everydayhealth.com/wellness/united-states-of-stress/link-between-stress-inflammation/

2 https://bebrainfit.com/vitamins-anxiety-stress/

3 https://www.prevention.com/health/memory/a20462907/mindfulness-meditation-slows-progression-of-alzheimers-and-dementia/

4 https://www.medicalnewstoday.com/articles/310148#Visual-spatial-memory-improvements-greater-for-yoga-meditation-group

5 https://www.mayoclinic.org/healthy-lifestyle/stress-management/in-depth/exercise-and-stress/art-20044469

6 https://www.ncbi.nlm.nih.gov/pmc/articles/PMC3734071/

7 https://www.psypost.org/2019/02/listening-to-the-music-you-love-will-make-your-brain-release-more-dopamine-study-finds

8 https://brainmd.com/blog/relax-your-mind-with-gaba/

9 https://nootriment.com/lemon-balm/

10 https://www.curejoy.com/content/ashwagandha-for-stress/

11 https://pubmed.ncbi.nlm.nih.gov/26974233/

Chapter 9

1 https://www.sciencedaily.com/releases/2018/05/180517113856.htm

2 https://www.psychologytoday.com/us/blog/the-antidepressant-diet/201706/social-loneliness-may- make-the-depressed-even-more-so

3   https://aginginplace.org/isolation-induced-depression-in-seniors/

4   https://www.ncoa.org/wp-content/uploads/Depression_Older_Persons_
    FactSheet_2009.pdf

5   https://www.apa.org/news/press/releases/2017/08/lonely-die

6   https://www.tandfonline.com/doi/abs/10.1080/13607863.2011.628977

7   https://jech.bmj.com/content/66/8/730

8   https://www.bmj.com/content/339/bmj.b2462

Chapter 10

1   https://www.cambridge.org/core/journals/the-british-journal-of-psychiatry/article/
    latelife-depression-and-risk-of-vascular-dementia-and-alzheimers-disease-systematic-
    review-and-metaanalysis-of-communitybased-cohort-studies/8944E89B957C
    C6BF6499A5A750614442

2   https://www.ncbi.nlm.nih.gov/pmc/articles/PMC3122998/

3   https://link.springer.com/article/10.1007/s11064-007-9385-y

4   https://www.tandfonline.com/doi/abs/10.1080/00048670802534408

5   https://pubmed.ncbi.nlm.nih.gov/28668539/

6   https://bmcmedicine.biomedcentral.com/articles/10.1186/s12916-017-0791-y#Sec18

7   https://journals.plos.org/plosone/article?id=10.1371/journal.pone.0016268

8   https://www.healthline.com/health/depression/cognitive-behavioral-therapy

9   https://www.health.com/condition/depression/types-of-meditation-for-depression

10 https://www.ncbi.nlm.nih.gov/pmc/articles/PMC2412901/

11 https://medicalxpress.com/news/2018-06-link-antidepressant-treatment-resistance-
    inflammation.html

12 https://www.healthline.com/health-news/certain-antidepressants-linked-to-
    increased-dementia-risk#2

13 https://alz-journals.onlinelibrary.wiley.com/doi/full/10.1002/alz.12113

14 https://www.bmj.com/content/345/bmj.e6231

15 https://www.webmd.com/alzheimers/news/20170330/drug-tied-to-dementia-risk-
    overprescribed-to-seniors-study#1

16 https://www.ncbi.nlm.nih.gov/pmc/articles/PMC5907560/

17 https://www.sciencedaily.com/releases/2018/07/180719112024.htm

18 https://www.alz.co.uk/news/smoking-increases-risk-of-dementia

19 https://www.alzheimers.org.uk/news/2018-05-03/aaic-lancet-commission-reveals-t
    hird-cases-dementia-may-be-preventable-alzheimers

20 https://www.ncbi.nlm.nih.gov/pmc/articles/PMC3647614/

21 https://apps.who.int/iris/bitstream/handle/10665/128041/WHO_NMH_PND_CIC_TKS_14.1_eng.pdf;jsessionid=298266DEA7FCC8FDABFCDF747C90BF6B?sequence=1

22 https://pubs.niaaa.nih.gov/publications/arh25-4/299-306.htm

23 https://www.webmd.com/alzheimers/news/20110817/moderate-alcohol-drinking-may-cut-alzheimers-risk#1

24 https://www.hear-it.org/hearing-loss-may-lead-depression

25 https://www.healthyhearing.com/report/52548-New-research-links-hearing-loss-to-an-increased-risk-of-falls

26 https://katekunkel.com/blog/f/our-gut-depression-and-alzheimer

27 https://pubmed.ncbi.nlm.nih.gov/23337978/

28 https://www.livescience.com/36108-cognitive-simulation-alzheimers-disease.html

29 https://www.mayoclinic.org/diseases-conditions/hearing-loss/symptoms-causes/syc-20373072

30 https://www.aarp.org/health/conditions-treatments/info-2017/inexpensive-hearing-aids-safe-fd.html

31 https://www.amazon.com/s?k=sound+amplification+device&ref=nb_sb_noss_2

32 https://www.newsmax.com/Health/Health-News/vision-loss-cognitive-decline/2017/08/24/id/809499/

33 https://jamanetwork.com/journals/jamaophthalmology/article-abstract/2764384

34 https://www.health.harvard.edu/pain/posture-and-back-health

35 https://greatist.com/health/ultimate-guide-good-posture#7

36 https://pubmed.ncbi.nlm.nih.gov/17224578/

37 https://www.ncbi.nlm.nih.gov/pmc/articles/PMC6153553/

38 https://psychcentral.com/news/2019/10/30/early-retirement-can-accelerate-cognitive-decline/151461.html

Chapter 12

1 https://www.prevention.com/food-nutrition/healthy-eating/a26873528/dirty-dozen-foods-2019/

2 https://www.ncbi.nlm.nih.gov/pmc/articles/PMC6110503/

3 https://pubmed.ncbi.nlm.nih.gov/23850343/

4 https://www.longevitylive.com/health-living/garlic-health-benefits-brain/

5 https://pubmed.ncbi.nlm.nih.gov/16484570/

6 https://www.webmd.com/vitamins/ai/ingredientmono-450/fructo-oligosaccharides-fos

7 https://pubmed.ncbi.nlm.nih.gov/22771051/

8   https://www.ncbi.nlm.nih.gov/books/NBK10807/

9   https://www.amenclinics.com/conditions/adhd-add/

10   https://pubmed.ncbi.nlm.nih.gov/25748372/

11   https://news.nus.edu.sg/research/mushrooms-reduce-cognitive-decline

12   https://www.ncbi.nlm.nih.gov/pmc/articles/PMC5216880/

13   https://www.medicalnewstoday.com/articles/301506

14   https://www.sciencedirect.com/science/article/pii/S2352939317300623

15   https://www.ncbi.nlm.nih.gov/pmc/articles/PMC4387064/

16   https://www.webmd.com/healthy-aging/news/20120426/berries-may-slow-memory-loss#1

17   https://academic.oup.com/ajcn/article/101/3/538/4569408

18   https://draxe.com/nutrition/plantains/

19   https://www.cambridge.org/core/journals/british-journal-of-nutrition/article/concord-grape-juice-supplementation-improves-memory-function-in-older-adults-with-mild-cognitive-impairment/FC419D32F0D6A023EAAF54E811252D16

20   https://academic.oup.com/biomedgerontology/article/71/12/1596/2513764

21   https://biox.stanford.edu/highlight/caffeine-may-counter-age-related-inflammation

22   https://www.health.harvard.edu/alzheimers-and-dementia/regular-tea-drinking-linked-with-dementia-prevention

23   https://www.liebertpub.com/doi/10.1089/jmf.2009.1374

24   https://www.sciencedirect.com/science/article/abs/pii/S0963996917301941

25   https://psychcentral.com/news/2020/02/01/antioxidant-in-fruits-vegetables-tea-linked-to-lower-risk-of-alzheimers/153870.html

26   https://www.cbc.ca/marketplace/blog/full-tea-test-results

27   https://pubmed.ncbi.nlm.nih.gov/15814269/

28   https://www.sciencedaily.com/releases/2012/04/120422162217.htm

29   https://www.greenmedinfo.com/article/medium-chain-triglycerides-coconut-fat-increase-cognitive-performance-alzheime

30   https://pubmed.ncbi.nlm.nih.gov/24150106/

31   https://www.youtube.com/watch?v=Dfux-5Z4COo&feature=youtu.be

32   https://www.ncbi.nlm.nih.gov/pmc/articles/PMC3405188/

33   https://pubmed.ncbi.nlm.nih.gov/22005283/

34   https://pubmed.ncbi.nlm.nih.gov/23466052/

35   https://www.cambridge.org/core/journals/nutrition-research-reviews/article/phenolic-compounds-of-olive-oil-structure-biological-activity-and-beneficial-effects-on-human-health/EE4FA28B6CD751AA15B278589A447A3D

36   https://pubmed.ncbi.nlm.nih.gov/12550060/

37   https://pubmed.ncbi.nlm.nih.gov/23850343/

38   https://journals.plos.org/plosone/article?id=10.1371/journal.pone.0016268

39   https://www.consumerhealthdigest.com/ingredients/carbohydrates.html

40   https://www.ncbi.nlm.nih.gov/pmc/articles/PMC6567199/

41   https://dontwastethecrumbs.com/ways-use-flaxseed/

42   https://www.nutrition-and-you.com/pumpkin-seeds.html

43   https://pubmed.ncbi.nlm.nih.gov/27348418/

44   https://pubmed.ncbi.nlm.nih.gov/24315808/

45   https://pubmed.ncbi.nlm.nih.gov/26846140/

46   https://pubmed.ncbi.nlm.nih.gov/29017372/

47   https://www.onegreenplanet.org/natural-health/how-cashews-can-help-with-stress-and-anxiety/

48   https://www.onegreenplanet.org/natural-health/how-your-food-choices-impact-your-hormones/

49   https://pubmed.ncbi.nlm.nih.gov/22458696/

50   https://www.webmd.com/food-recipes/benefits-pistachios#1

51   https://www.researchgate.net/publication/7768753_Walnut_Extract_Inhibits_the_Fibrillization_of_Amyloid_Beta-Protein_and_also_Defibrillizes_its_Preformed_Fibrils

52   https://link.springer.com/article/10.1007/s12603-014-0569-2

53   https://downshiftology.com/5-things-you-need-to-know-about-cassava-flour/

54   https://foodrevolution.org/blog/health-benefits-of-curcumin

55   https://www.greenmedinfo.com/blog/5-most-powerful-health-benefits-ginger

56   https://www.healthline.com/health/diabetes/ginger-and-diabetes#benefits

57   https://www.healthline.com/health/ginger-for-arthritis#research

58   https://www.ars.usda.gov/news-events/news/research-news/2009/researchers-study-effect-of-cinnamon-compounds-on-brain-cells/

59   https://www.researchgate.net/publication/232240488_Oregano_Overview_of_the_Literature_on_Health_Benefits

60   https://www.ncbi.nlm.nih.gov/pmc/articles/PMC5242351/

61   https://www.sciencedirect.com/science/article/abs/pii/S0378874105003983

62   https://europepmc.org/article/MED/12209371/

63   https://pubmed.ncbi.nlm.nih.gov/27527000/

64   https://www.hindawi.com/journals/ecam/2016/2680409/

65   https://www.sciencedirect.com/science/article/abs/pii/S000629520800292X

66   https://pubmed.ncbi.nlm.nih.gov/21877951/

67   https://pubmed.ncbi.nlm.nih.gov/12605619/

68 https://journals.sagepub.com/doi/abs/10.1177/0895937409335642

69 https://pubmed.ncbi.nlm.nih.gov/29422459/

70 https://pubmed.ncbi.nlm.nih.gov/7024026/

Chapter 13

1 https://www.drweil.com/diet-nutrition/cooking-cookware/cooking-to-fight-inflammation/

2 https://www.cambridge.org/core/journals/journal-of-nutritional-science/article/dietary-patterns-are-associated-with-cognitive-function-in-the-reasons-for-geographic-and-racial-differences-in-stroke-regards-cohort/B7612048AF9A363A41C6B740FA1FB7EE

3 https://www.cambridge.org/core/journals/journal-of-nutritional-science/article/dietary-patterns-are-associated-with-cognitive-function-in-the-reasons-for-geographic-and-racial-differences-in-stroke-regards-cohort/B7612048AF9A363A41C6B740FA1FB7EE

4 https://www.clinicalnutritionjournal.com/article/S0261-5614(16)00035-2/fulltext

5 https://www.sciencedirect.com/science/article/pii/S0197458014003480

6 https://www.academia.edu/13789040/Alcohol_consumption_in_mild_cognitive_impairment_and_dementia_harmful_or_neuroprotective?email_work_card=view-paper

7 https://pubs.niaaa.nih.gov/publications/aa63/aa63.htm

8 https://globalhealing.com/natural-health/how-alcohol-affects-the-gut-microbiome/#references

9 https://pubmed.ncbi.nlm.nih.gov/12636463/

10 https://www.rt.com/news/479111-soybean-oil-change-mice-brain/

11 https://pubmed.ncbi.nlm.nih.gov/15735094/

12 https://medicalxpress.com/news/2017-12-canola-oil-linked-worsened-memory.html

13 https://www.resourcesforlife.com/docs/item1225

14 https://www.organicconsumers.org/news/glyphosate-roundup-disrupt-gut-microbiome-contradicting-regulators-assuptions

Chapter 14

1 https://drjockers.com/category/health-news/fasting/

2 https://pubmed.ncbi.nlm.nih.gov/21527899/

3 https://www.sciencedirect.com/science/article/pii/S193152441400200X

4   https://www.ncbi.nlm.nih.gov/pmc/articles/PMC4013772/

5   https://pubmed.ncbi.nlm.nih.gov/12558961/

6   https://pubmed.ncbi.nlm.nih.gov/21898045/

7   https://www.medicalnewstoday.com/articles/320101

8   https://www.ncbi.nlm.nih.gov/pmc/articles/PMC3919445/

9   https://www.ncbi.nlm.nih.gov/pmc/articles/PMC6137621/

10   https://www.sciencedirect.com/science/article/pii/S0022282818303584

11   https://www.sciencedirect.com/science/article/pii/S0969996119303900

12   https://www.dietdoctor.com/the-hidden-truth-behind-ancel-keys-famous-fat-graph

Chapter 15

1   https://www.pnas.org/content/110/23/9523

2   https://stemcellstransplantinstitute.com/2019/06/09/vitamin-c-and-alzheimers-disease/

3   https://www.mayoclinic.org/diseases-conditions/alzheimers-disease/expert-answers/vitamin-d-alzheimers/faq-20111272

4   https://www.verywellhealth.com/why-is-vitamin-d-so-important-to-thyroid-patients-3232755

5   https://www.medscape.com/viewarticle/839763

6   https://www.researchgate.net/profile/David_Hanley2/publication/8061054_Vitamin_D_Insufficiency_in_North_America/links/00b7d5265888a11eb200 0000/Vitamin-D-Insufficiency-in-North-America.pdf?origin=publication_detail

7   https://www.newhope.com/science/vitamin-e-may-reduce-alzheimers-risk

8   https://academic.oup.com/ajcn/article/77/4/975/4689775

9   https://pubmed.ncbi.nlm.nih.gov/29794977/

10   https://www.webmd.com/alzheimers/news/20160818/calcium-supplements-might-raise-older-womens-dementia-risk#1

11   https://pubmed.ncbi.nlm.nih.gov/31685499/

12   https://www.researchgate.net/publication/303768692_Erythrocyte_intracellular_Mg2_concentration_as_an_index_of_recognition_and_memory

13   https://www.ncbi.nlm.nih.gov/pmc/articles/PMC4790399/

14   https://www.naturalhealth365.com/coq10-dementia-2006.html

15   https://www.ncbi.nlm.nih.gov/pmc/articles/PMC2785862/

16   http://www.dartmouth.edu/~rswenson/NeuroSci/chapter_11.html

17   https://www.ncbi.nlm.nih.gov/pmc/articles/PMC3286229/

18   https://pubmed.ncbi.nlm.nih.gov/17998483/

19   https://www.drperlmutter.com/daily-dose-dha/

Chapter 16

1   https://qbi.uq.edu.au/brain-basics/brain-physiology/what-neurogenesis
2   https://www.psychologytoday.com/us/basics/neuroplasticity
3   http://longevity.stanford.edu/a-consensus-on-the-brain-training-industry-from-the-scientific-community-2/

Chapter 17

1   https://www.ncbi.nlm.nih.gov/pmc/articles/PMC4087081/
2   https://www.youtube.com/watch?v=Fo0K_n3VLG4&list=PL8613AD2409CFDE4E
3   https://www.youtube.com/watch?v=Y1-Apl0Zi2Q
4   https://www.psychologytoday.com/intl/blog/your-musical-self/201101/why-listening-music-makes-us-feel-good
5   https://www.aarp.org/health/healthy-living/info-2018/live-music-longevity-happiness-fd.html
6   https://www.hsrd.research.va.gov/news/research_news/music-010614.cfm
7   https://flavourjournal.biomedcentral.com/articles/10.1186/2044-7248-3-9

Chapter 18

1   https://pubmed.ncbi.nlm.nih.gov/25544932/
2   https://www.youtube.com/watch?v=R0JKCYZ8hng
3   https://www.sciencedirect.com/topics/neuroscience/neuroplasticity
4   https://www.newscientist.com/article/dn28266-musicians-brains-fire-symmetrically-when-they-listen-to-music/
5   https://www.psychologytoday.com/us/blog/the-athletes-way/201406/does-playing-musical-instrument-make-you-smarter
6   https://www.livescience.com/7950-music-improves-brain-function.html
7   https://www.collective-evolution.com/2019/12/10/research-shows-we-can-heal-with-vibration-frequency-sound/
8   https://www.greenmedinfo.com/article/improved-executive-function-and-callosal-white-matter-microstructure-after-rhy
9   https://www.respectfulbeats.com/blogs/

10 https://www.abc.net.au/classic/features/how-music-works-what-happens-to-your-brain-when-you-sing/10115596

11 https://www.sciencedaily.com/releases/2017/12/171221101402.htm

12 https://pubmed.ncbi.nlm.nih.gov/15669447/

13 https://www.bbc.com/news/science-environment-23230411

14 http://alzheimersprevention.org/research/12-minute-memory-exercise/

15 https://www.dailymail.co.uk/health/article-4581438/Why-elderly-prescribed-ballroom-dancing.html

16 https://www.healthy-holistic-living.com/dancing-can-reverse-the-signs-of-aging-in-the-brain

17 https://www.awakeningfromalzheimers.com/this-may-be-the-most-powerful-way-to-a-stronger-brain/

18 https://www.youtube.com/channel/UCyZKmU60yoTKDChV-WnWPnw

19 https://www.tandfonline.com/doi/full/10.1080/07421656.2016.1166832

Chapter 19

1 https://www.prohealth.com/library/frankincense-food-for-a-happy-brain-and-neurological-system-42759

2 https://journals.sagepub.com/doi/10.1177/2045125312436573

3 https://scienzaonline.org/scienceonline-news/item/1443-rosemary-aroma-can-aid-children-s-working-memory.html

4 https://www.scirp.org/journal/paperinformation.aspx?paperid=86207

5 https://naturallivingfamily.com/essential-oils-for-stress/

6 https://naturallivingfamily.com/best-essential-oils-for-depression/

7 https://www.ncbi.nlm.nih.gov/pmc/articles/PMC3612440/

8 https://naturallivingfamily.com/best-essential-oils-for-sleep/

9 https://pubmed.ncbi.nlm.nih.gov/22475718/

10 https://www.ncbi.nlm.nih.gov/pmc/articles/PMC3924999/

11 https://bebrainfit.com/gaba-neurotransmitter/

12 https://www.themiracleofessentialoils.com/essential-oils-for-leaky-gut-syndrome/

13 https://lindseyelmore.com/essential-oils-for-gut-health/

14 https://wellnessmama.com/404091/ice-bath-benefits/

15 https://www.ncbi.nlm.nih.gov/pmc/articles/PMC6802936/

16 https://www.quietmindfdn.org/blog/photobiomodulation-for-alzheimers-disease

17 https://www.quietmindfdn.org/equipment.html

18 https://katekunkel.com/vibroacoustic-therapy

19 https://www.quora.com/Do-YouTube-videos-about-brain-waves-really-help-Are-there-studies-that-prove-they-are-effective-How-effective-are-they-and-to-what-degree

20 https://pubmed.ncbi.nlm.nih.gov/28739482/

21 https://www.ncbi.nlm.nih.gov/pmc/articles/PMC6130417/

22 http://www.bartelcameronassoc.com/dr-lee-bartel.htm

23 https://www.soundoasis.com/products/sleep-sound-therapy-systems/vibroacoustic-therapy-system/

24 https://holistichealthscience.com/

25 https://www.dementiacarecentral.com/aboutdementia/treating/cbd/

26 https://www.sciencedirect.com/science/article/pii/B9780128120125000318?via%3Dihub

27 https://drjockers.com/hyperbaric-oxygen-therapy/

Chapter 20

1   https://pubmed.ncbi.nlm.nih.gov/26168376/

2   https://www.ncbi.nlm.nih.gov/pmc/articles/PMC3004979/

3   https://www.everydayhealth.com/alternative-health/living-with/ways-practice-breath-focused-meditation/

4   https://www.healthline.com/health/exercise-fitness/tai-chi-moves

5   https://www.yogajournal.com/yoga-101/what-is-qi-gong

6   https://www.yogajournal.com/yoga-101

7   https://www.webmd.com/balance/guide/transcendental-meditation-benefits-technique

8   https://www.healthstatus.com/health_blog/what-is-dementia/effect-positive-attitude/

9   https://www.ajc.com/lifestyles/study-links-repeated-negative-thinking-increased-risk-dementia/

10 https://www.ncbi.nlm.nih.gov/pmc/articles/PMC4853823/

11 https://alz-journals.onlinelibrary.wiley.com/doi/full/10.1002/alz.12116

About the Author

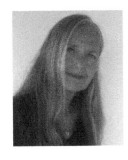

Kate Kunkel is a harpist who has nurtured the healing power of music and shared its power through workshops and coaching and in her first book, *The Healing Sound of Music*.

When her mom was diagnosed with dementia in 2010, a whole new dimension was added to Kate's life, and she embarked on a mission to research and study this terrible disease in an effort to ensure she did not follow the path her mother was taking.

What Kate learned inspired her to make serious lifestyle modifications, including switching to a whole-foods, plant-based diet and training as a vegan nutritionist and health coach. The changes that Kate instituted herself became a program that she now shares with clients who are also determined to maintain optimal brain function and enjoy a healthier, more vibrant life.

In personal coaching sessions, in the "Eight Weeks to a Better Brain" group program, in her blog, and now in this book, Kate has one simple mission: To spread the word that dementia is largely a preventable disease, and that it is never too early to protect your brain. But it can get too late.

Kate lives on a quiet retreat property on the coast of Ecuador with her husband, Lynn, and five rescue cats.

Connect with Kate, read the blog and learn about the programs at her website: KateKunkel.com

Made in United States
Orlando, FL
16 June 2022

18875623R00167